Nutrition and Well-being for Vulnerable Adults

Underpinning knowledge for frontline workers in adult social care

Malcolm Day, Alison Smith and Lisa-Jayne Cruickshank

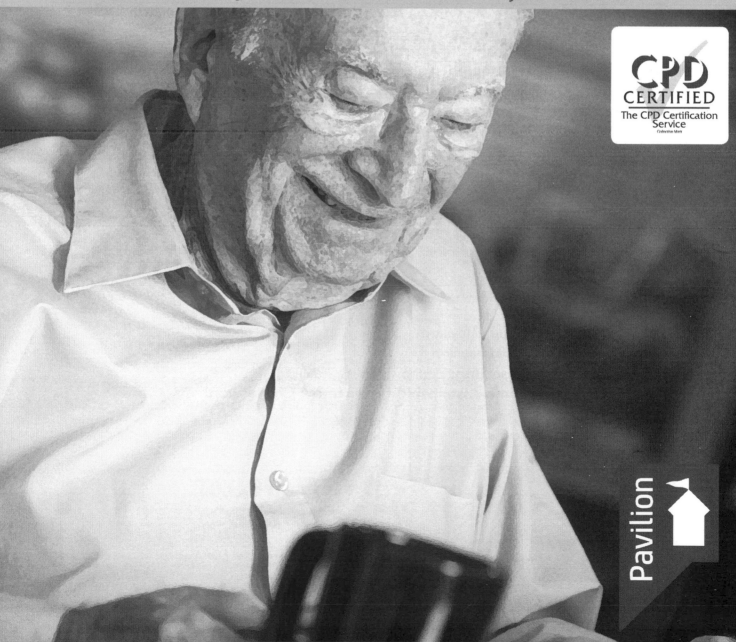

Pavilion

Chapter four

About the authors

Malcolm Day is a registered nurse and practice educator. He is a Fellow of the Institute for Learning and a Fellow of the Higher Education Academy. Malcolm has previously worked as a clinical lead in care of older people, and as a care home manager. He has held university lectureships in nursing, community care, and care management. Malcolm is currently a lecturer in adult nursing at the University of Nottingham. He is author of *Caring for the Older Person*, *Safeguarding Vulnerable Adults*, *Caring for the Person with Dementia*, *Support People at the End of Life* and co-author of *Supporting People in their Own Homes*, also published by Pavilion.

Alison Smith qualified as a registered dietitian in 1996 and has worked in the community in Peterborough since 1998. Since 2001 Alison has specialised in prevention and treatment of malnutrition in older adults in the community and care homes, and in adults with progressive neurological disorders. Alison has been public relations officer for the Nutrition Advisory Group for Older People (NAGE), a specialist group of the British Dietetic Association (BDA), since 2009, a post she also held between 2003 and 2007, and as such has spoken at national conferences, written a number of journal articles and been involved in several national initiatives to combat malnutrition in older people.

Lisa-Jayne Cruickshank qualified as a registered dietitian in 2000. She has specialised in working with older adults since 2004, both in hospitals and in the community. She is now working in a community dietetic post in Warwickshire. Lisa-Jayne recently completed a postgraduate diploma in gerontology at King's College, London, and has previously worked with NAGE.

About this training resource

In January 2011 NVQs in Health and Social Care were replaced with the new Level 2 and 3 Diplomas in Health and Social Care. The new QCF qualifications provide a 'mix and match' approach to meeting the different training and development needs of the social care workforce.

There are now three types of qualification:

- Award (1–12 credits)
- Certificate (13–36 credits)
- Diploma (above 36 credits) – not linked to the 14–19 Diploma.

Every unit within these qualifications has a credit value and a level.

- One credit represents 10 hours of average learning time, so the credit value reflects approximately how much time the unit takes to complete.
- The level shows how difficult the unit or qualification is (from entry level to level 8).

From September 2011, qualifications in food safety and nutrition include:

- **Level 2 Award in Food Safety in Health and Social Care and Early Years and Childcare Settings:** This is a qualification for people working in health and social care who are completing their initial training in food safety.
- **Level 2 Award in Promoting Food Safety and Nutrition in Health and Social Care or Early Years and Childcare Settings:** This qualification will assess the competence of learners working in any health and social care setting in which diet and nutrition is particularly important.

This training resource draws upon the previous work undertaken by Skills for Care to identify underpinning knowledge for the nutrition and well-being knowledge set. This previous work has underpinned the development of the new qualifications in food safety and nutrition, and includes materials on:

- preparing and presenting food to service users
- roles and boundaries
- nutrition and well-being
- legislation and guidance related to food and drink.

These materials cover the underpinning knowledge for the following mandatory and optional units of the new Level 2 awards in food safety and nutrition:

- HSC 2029: Meet Food Safety Requirements when Providing Food and Drink for Individuals
- HSC 2014: Support Individuals to Eat and Drink
- FSN 201: Contribute to Promoting Nutrition and Hydration in Health and Social Care Settings
- FSN 301: Promote Nutrition and Hydration in Health and Social Care Settings

These materials will also be of value to new workers entering the social care sector, as well as social care workers who are continually developing their knowledge to assist vulnerable people with their nutrition and well-being.

Throughout this training resource there are ☺ learning activities for you to complete, which introduce you to the key aspects that are going to be covered.

You should complete these before you start or continue your reading and discuss them with a colleague or your supervisor. At the end of each chapter there is a quiz to help you revise the knowledge that has been covered. The answers to the quizzes are provided in **Appendix A**.

At the end of each chapter, there is also a continuing professional development (CPD) log ✍ for you to complete with your supervisor. This is particularly important if you intend to undertake the new nutrition and well-being qualifications as you can be given credit for any prior learning you have undertaken – based on the content, number of hours and level of study you have completed.

The CPD log will also assist your manager to keep a record of your training, which is a requirement of your social care inspectorate and the Care Quality Commission.

Chapter one

Preparing and presenting food to service users

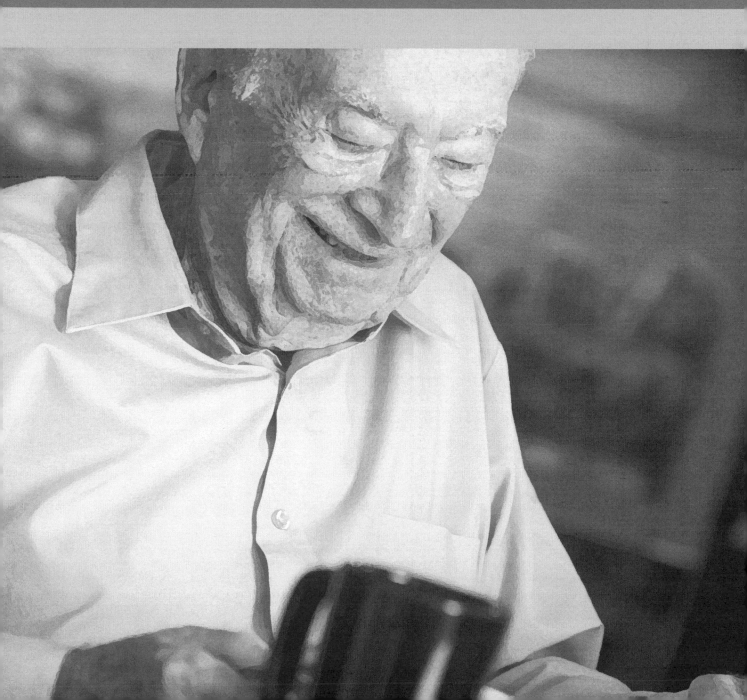

Chapter one

Preparing and presenting food to service users

☺ Key learning activity

This activity will provide you with key background information before you read **Chapter one**. It draws on information provided by the NHS Choices *Live Well* webpage, in relation to:

- healthy diet

- ages and stages

- health issues.

The website you need to access for this activity is www.nhs.uk/livewell/healthy-eating/Pages/Healthyeating.aspx

Make a note of your answers and discuss these with a colleague or your supervisor before you start your reading.

Q1. Click on 'Food and diet'.
- What are the eight tips for a healthy diet?

Q2. Click on 'A balanced diet'.
- What are the five main food groups?

Q3. Click on 'Fat: the facts'.
- What is the difference between saturated and unsaturated fat?

Q4. Click on 'Men's health 60-plus' and take a look at 'Eat well over 60'.
- What can older people do to ensure a healthy and nutritious diet?

AIMS OF THE CHAPTER

At the end of this chapter, the learner will have considered:

- the factors that may affect the dietary requirements of individuals, for example, age, culture, religion, medical conditions, the availability of food etc

- the importance of appropriate preparation and presentation of food and drink, for example, attractiveness, consistency, temperature, variety etc

- the importance of creating an appropriate environment in which to eat and drink, for example, the use of eating aids, choice of menu, environment etc.

This chapter covers the underpinning knowledge for the following Level 2 mandatory and optional units in food safety and nutrition (the number following the unit number refers to a specific learning outcome):

- HSC 2014:1

- HSC 2014:2

- HSC 2014:3

- FSN 201:1

- FSN 201:7

- FSN 301:1

- FSN 301:2

- FSN 301:3

FACTORS AFFECTING THE DIETARY REQUIREMENTS OF INDIVIDUALS

Age, culture, religion, medical conditions, personal choice and the availability of food can all influence our dietary requirements. A well balanced diet should contain enough of the following nutrients to meet our daily needs:

- protein from meat, fish, dairy products, beans and pulses

- carbohydrate from bread, potatoes, pasta, rice and cereals

- fats from oily fish, nuts and seeds, margarine, olive oil and sunflower oil

- minerals, for example, calcium for strong bones

- vitamins, for example, vitamin K for blood clotting

- water.

A proper balance of these nutrients is very important. This can be achieved by having the right proportions of the food groups in the diet, as illustrated by the eatwell plate on the NHS Choices Live Well webpages at www.nhs.uk/livewell/goodfood/pages/eatwell-plate.aspx

Recent evidence in the UK has shown how food excesses – particularly an excess of fat – can contribute to obesity, increased risk of heart disease and some types of cancer. So what is a healthy diet?

The NHS Choices Live Well webpage www.nhs.uk/LiveWell/healthy-eating/Pages/Healthyeating.aspx identifies eight tips for making healthier dietary choices.

1. **Meals should be based on starchy foods.** Starchy foods should make up about a third of the food we eat. Wholegrain varieties, such as wholemeal bread, whole wheat pasta, brown rice and wholegrain breakfast cereals, contain more fibre than white or refined starchy foods. They are digested more slowly, so they make us feel full for longer.

2. **Eat more fruit and vegetables.** The NHS Live Well webpage advises that people eat at least five portions of a variety of fruit and vegetables every day. One portion of fruit and vegetables is 80g; this is roughly equivalent to one apple, banana, pear, orange or other similar sized fruit, or a 150ml glass of fruit juice.

3. **Eat more fish.** Fish contains many vitamins and minerals and is a good source of protein. We should aim to eat two portions of fish a week, including one portion of oily fish. Oily fish contains omega 3 fatty acids, which are good for the heart. Oily fish include salmon, mackerel, trout, herring, fresh tuna, sardines, pilchards and eel.

4. **Cut down on saturated fat and sugar.** Too much saturated fat can increase blood cholesterol. Foods that are high in saturated fat include meat pies, sausages, meat with visible white fat, hard cheese, butter and lard, pastry, cakes and biscuits, and cream. Too much refined sugar can contribute to obesity and tooth decay. Foods that are high in refined sugar include sweetened beverages, sugary cereals, and sweet snacks such as biscuits and cakes.

5. **Eat less salt.** Too much salt can increase your blood pressure. People with high blood pressure have an increased risk of developing heart disease. A high salt content is more than 1.5g salt per 100g (or 0.6g sodium). A low salt content is 0.3g salt or less per 100g (or 0.1g sodium).

6. **Drink plenty of water.** We should drink at least six to eight glasses (1.2–1.6 litres) of water (or other fluids) every day. When the weather is warm or we are physically active, our bodies need more than this. It is important to note that some soft drinks are high in added sugar so diet or sugar-free varieties may be a better option.

7. **Do not miss breakfast.** Breakfast gives us the energy we need to face the day, as well as some of the vitamins and minerals we need for good health. Research shows that eating breakfast can actually help people control their weight. The NHS Live Well website recommends a nutritious breakfast, such as a bowl of wholegrain cereal with some sliced banana, for a healthy start to the day.

8. **Be active and try to be a healthy weight.** When we need to lose a little weight, the key points to remember are: control portion size, choose low fat and low sugar foods, and eat plenty of fruit and vegetables. Becoming more active promotes weight loss and helps to maintain a healthy weight. Individuals who want to become more active need to gradually build up the amount of exercise they do every day, for example, walking to work rather than catching the bus, taking the stairs instead of a lift, or going for a regular walk.

HOW AGE AFFECTS DIETARY REQUIREMENTS

The dietary needs of an individual will often change throughout their life. For example, a diet suitable for an adolescent may not be right for an older person. This section will help you to understand and appreciate how dietary needs change across a person's lifespan.

Infancy

When a baby is born its digestive system is immature and unable to digest most foods. It is for this reason that a baby's nutritional needs are met entirely by milk. Breast milk is the best source of nutrition for newborn babies, as it provides easily digestible nutrients in the right quantities. Breastfed babies are at less risk of stomach upsets and ear, respiratory and urinary tract infections. They are also less likely to experience constipation and vomiting. (See www.nhs.uk/Planners/ breastfeeding/Pages/why-breastfeed.aspx for more information.) Alternatives to human milk are modified infant formulas, which must meet European standards for nutritional composition. However, they cannot fully reproduce all of the components of breast milk. It is essential that the formula is made up according to the instructions on the container to ensure the baby gains the correct weight. Strict hygiene precautions are also required when preparing the feed, in order to kill any harmful bacteria that may be present.

Weaning

The Department of Health in the UK recommends starting solid foods around the age of six months (see www.nhs.uk/Planners/birthtofive/Pages/Weaningfirststeps.aspx). Recent evidence indicates that babies should start weaning by six months of age but not before four months (17 weeks). By six months, a baby's nutritional requirements can no longer be met by milk alone and the digestive system has matured enough to cope with solid food. The aim of weaning is to gradually introduce a variety of tastes and textures so that, by the age of one, the baby is enjoying a varied and healthy diet. Weaning is usually carried out in three main stages.

- **Stage one (by six months but not before four months):** The baby should start taking food from a spoon and moving food from the front to the back of the mouth for swallowing. Once the baby is used to taking food from a spoon, the amount and number of times a day that food is offered should be gradually increased. Examples of stage one weaning foods include puréed non-fibrous vegetables or soft fruit mixed with either breast milk or formula.

- **Stage two (six to nine months):** During stage two the baby should start chewing soft lumps, self-feeding using their hands and sipping fluids from a cup. Examples of stage two weaning foods include mashed meat, fish, vegetables or pasta and soft finger foods, for example, fruit and cooked vegetables.

- **Stage three (nine to 12 months):** At this stage the baby may be self-feeding with a spoon. Foods should be mashed and chopped rather than puréed. The baby may also enjoy hard finger foods, such as chopped fruit, breadsticks or toast. Chewing these will help to develop the baby's facial muscles, which are important for speech. Babies should never be left alone while they are trying hard foods or feeding themselves, due to the risk of choking.

During weaning it is important to offer a variety of foods to ensure that the baby receives all the necessary vitamins and minerals. A baby should have around 500ml of breast milk or formula a day, until they are well established on solids. By one year of age, aim to include three meals a day, each containing one serving of starchy food, a fruit and a vegetable, and one to two servings per day of protein-rich food such as soft cooked meat, fish or pulses.

Vitamin drops

Vitamin drops should be given to all babies from six months of age if they are breastfed or if formula milk intake is less than 500ml day.

Foods to be avoided

■ **Salt/spices:** Do not add them to food or give salty foods, for example, crisps. A small amount of mild spices, for example, coriander and cumin, can be used for older babies.

■ **Sugar:** Adding sugar to foods should be limited to that needed for tart or sour stewed fruit.

■ **Foods containing gluten (wheat, rye, barley, oats):** Wait until six months (26 weeks) of age before giving rusks, bread, cereals or biscuits.

■ **Milk and milk products:** Formula or breast milk is best used for drinks until the baby is one year old. Whole cow's milk can be used in cooking after six months (26 weeks) of age, for example, yogurts, fromage frais, custards, sauces and mixed with cereals. After one year whole cows milk can be used as a drink.

■ **Cheese:** Cheese can be introduced from six months of age. Start off with cottage cheese owing to the high salt content of hard cheeses.

■ **Honey:** Honey should not be given to babies under one year of age as it has been found to occasionally contain harmful spores.

■ **Nuts and seeds:** Whole nuts should not be given to babies and children under five years of age due to the risk of choking. Finely ground nuts, for example, smooth nut butters can be given from six months. If a baby has known allergies or a family risk of allergy, nuts should be avoided until three years of age.

■ **Eggs:** Eggs should not be introduced until six months of age. They must be well cooked until the white and yolk are hard, owing to the risk of *Salmonella* food poisoning.

■ **Shellfish:** Shellfish should not be given to babies under one year of age as they are associated with a high risk of food poisoning.

■ **Liver:** Liver is extremely high in vitamin A so should not be eaten before six months of age. After six months of age, limit liver intake to no more than once a week.

■ **Shark, swordfish and marlin:** Avoid giving these to babies under one year of age owing to the high mercury content.

From six months, water and diluted, unsweetened fruit juices (one part juice to 10 parts water) can be offered at mealtimes. Fizzy drinks, fruit squashes, tea, coffee or drinks with artificial sweeteners should not be given. Drinks between meals should be tap water, breast milk or formula. By one year, feeding from a bottle should be strongly discouraged as a cup is better for children's teeth.

Young children (one to four years)

Early childhood is an important time to complete the weaning process, reduce the amount of milk and establish good eating habits for life. A young child's energy and nutritional needs are high relative to their size; so their diet must be made up of small, regular and nutritionally dense meals. It is normal for a toddler's appetite to vary from day to day.

There are no specific recommendations for portion size in preschool children; rather, they should be allowed to eat according to their appetite. If the family diet is healthy, there is no need to rely on pre-prepared toddler food; children can have the same food as the rest of the family, which should include the following.

- **Starchy foods:** At least one serving of starchy carbohydrate, such as bread, rice, pasta, noodles, cereals or potatoes, with every meal.

- **Fruit and vegetables:** A child sized handful of fruit and vegetables about five times a day, for example, fruit in puddings or as snacks.

- **Milk and dairy foods:** Aim for three servings a day. A serving would be 120ml/4oz milk, a 120g pot of yoghurt, a slice of cheese or a serving of custard etc. Whole milk should be given to children under two years of age, semi-skimmed milk can be used for children over two years of age. Skimmed milk should not be used before five years of age.

- **Meat, fish and alternatives:** These should be eaten once or twice a day. Alternatives might include boiled eggs or pulses. Some types of fish, such as fresh tuna, king mackerel, swordfish and shark, should be avoided as they may contain high levels of mercury, which might affect a child's developing nervous system.

Fatty and sugary foods should not be given too often and, when they are, only in small amounts. Sugary foods and drinks (including fruit juice) can also significantly contribute to dental decay, especially when consumed between meals. Milk or water are the best drinks to have between meals.

The following nutrients are particularly important for preschool children.

- **Iron:** Requirements are relatively high but dietary intake is often low, especially if little or no meat is eaten. Foods rich in vitamin C will help the child to absorb iron from non-meat sources, for example, fresh orange juice taken with a meal. Deficiency is common in this age group.

- **Calcium:** Calcium is important for the healthy growth of bones and teeth. This requirement will usually be met if milk and other dairy products are taken daily as a regular part of the child's diet.

- **Vitamins A, C and D:** Vitamin A is needed for healthy skin and cell development and can often be lacking in diets within this age group. Vitamin C is important for the immune system and growth, and its intake may be low in children who don't eat many fruits or vegetables. Vitamin D is essential for the body's calcium metabolism and can be produced by the body when skin is exposed to sunlight during the summer months. The Department of Health recommends that children up to the age of five years of age, particularly from ethnic minority groups, are given a supplement of vitamins A, C and D (NHS Choices, b).

Primary and secondary school age children and young adults (five to 18 years)

Primary and secondary school age children still have high nutritional needs, and it is important that their meals and snacks continue to be rich in energy and nutrients. A variety of foods should be encouraged from each of the main food groups. School children's daily intake should focus on three regular meals a day, with any additional snacks eaten mid-morning, mid-afternoon or before bed. A healthy diet for an older child should include the following.

- **Starchy foods:** One portion of starchy carbohydrate at each meal and some snacks, for example, bread, rice, cereals, pasta, potatoes etc.

- **Fruit and vegetables:** A minimum of five portions of fruit and vegetables per day. A portion is the equivalent of a child's handful.

- **Milk and dairy foods:** Three servings of dairy foods per day. A serving would be one glass of milk (150–250ml), one 125g–150g pot of yogurt or fromage frais, a serving of cheese in a sandwich or on a pizza, a milk-based pudding, or a serving of tofu.

- **Meat, fish and alternatives:** Two servings per day or three servings for vegetarians. Fish should be offered twice per week and oily fish at least once per week. Examples of one serving are: 80–120g of meat or fish, two to four fish fingers, one to two eggs, or three to four tablespoons of pulses (depending on the age of the child).

- **Fatty and sugary foods:** Children should be encouraged to have healthy, nutritious snacks rather than lots of fatty and sugary foods and drinks.

- **Drinks:** Six to eight glasses per day are recommended.

For primary school age children the most recent diet and nutrition survey – *The National Diet and Nutrition Survey: Young people aged four to 18 years* (Gregory, 2000) – showed that zinc and vitamin A intakes are low for many children of primary school age.

Teenager's diets are commonly deficient in vitamin A, zinc, calcium, magnesium, iron, riboflavin and potassium. This is also a time when young people begin to develop independence from their parents and will want to make their own decisions about what food they eat. Teenagers' food choices are often governed by peer pressure or as an act of defiance against their parents.

Teenagers frequently skip breakfast but it is particularly important. A good breakfast can provide essential nutrients and improve concentration levels in the morning. The following nutrients are particularly important for school aged children.

- **Calcium** for healthy bone development. Good sources include dairy products like milk, cheese and yoghurt, as well as green leafy vegetables and cereals.

- **Folate** for growth. Good sources of folate include bread, green leafy vegetables, bananas and pulses.

- **Iron** helps to keep red blood cells healthy. Insufficient intake can lead to anaemia. Good sources of iron include red meat, pulses, liver and fortified breakfast cereals.

- **Zinc** for growth, healing and immune function. Good sources include meat, fish, eggs, cheese, nuts, wholegrain cereals and pulses.

- **Vitamin A** for growth and a healthy immune system. It is also associated with maintaining good vision in dim light. There are two forms of vitamin A: retinol found in animal foods, for example, liver, liver paté and eggs; and carotene found in fruit and vegetables, for example, carrots, sweet potato, mango, melon and apricots.

- **Magnesium** is important for development of the skeleton and nervous system. Good sources include cereals, green vegetables and nuts.

- **Riboflavin** is important for enabling the body to make use of energy. Good sources include cheese, milk, yoghurt, poultry, oily fish and eggs.

- **Potassium** regulates body fluids and blood pressure. Good sources include most fruit and vegetables.

Adults

Some risk factors for premature death in adults include:

- raised blood cholesterol

- raised blood pressure

- obesity and physical inactivity

- excessive alcohol intake.

The National Diet and Nutrition Survey: Adults aged 19 to 64, published in 2003, found that UK adults eat too much saturated fat, sugar and salt, and not enough dietary fibre – on average their fruit and vegetable intake is fewer than three portions a day. However, adults who eat a nutritious diet and are physically active can maintain a healthy body weight and reduce their risk of developing diet-related illnesses, such as type 2 diabetes, heart disease and some types of cancer.

Men in particular, should be wary of excess weight. In men, extra pounds tend to be stored around the abdomen. This increases their risk of developing heart disease and diabetes, to a greater extent than fat stored on the hips and thighs, which is more typical for women.

Pregnancy and breastfeeding place extra nutritional demands on women. Women are also at higher risk of developing iron deficiency anaemia than men. There may also be a link between alcohol consumption and certain diseases, such as breast cancer. Therefore, alcohol should not be consumed every day and, when it is consumed, women should not exceed two to three units of alcohol a day, and men no more than three to four. Healthy adults choosing a variety of foods from each of the food groups should not need a vitamin and mineral supplement. Research shows that people who eat at least five portions of fruit and vegetables a day have much lower rates of coronary heart disease and cancer.

Older adults

The nutritional needs of older adults can be difficult to categorise. This is because dietary needs depend on current health, and although many older people may be fit and active, some may be frail and require additional care. However, research shows that remaining active can help to maintain mental and physical health and independence, and preserve muscle tissue and mobility. Gardening, walking to the shops and housework all count as different types of physical activity.

Energy requirements can decline with age, particularly if physical activity is limited, but the need for protein, vitamins and minerals remains the same. It is vital that older people choose nutritionally dense food. This means that they need to eat a variety of foods to get all the vitamins and minerals they need, but with fewer calories (particularly if an individual is overweight or obese).

Older people who are obese should reduce their fat intake – particularly saturated fat – to maintain a healthy heart. However, fat reduction isn't appropriate if the person is frail, has lost weight, or has a very small appetite. Rather, additional fat intake may be required to increase the calories in meals and snacks to aid weight gain.

Older people can suffer from constipation and bowel problems. This can be due to reduced gut motility and inactivity, inadequate fluid intake, and the side effects of some medication. Eating high fibre cereal foods, and fruit and vegetables will help the gut to work properly. It is also important to drink plenty of fluid – at least six to eight medium size glasses a day.

Dehydration can make older people drowsy or confused. It is important to drink an adequate amount of fluid, even if this means extra trips to the toilet. The risk of dehydration can be higher in older people because their kidneys don't function as efficiently. Some older people are also not as sensitive to the feeling of thirst, while others restrict their own fluid intake as they are worried about being incontinent. Fluid intake doesn't just mean water; it can also include such drinks as tea, coffee, fruit juice and squash.

Fit and healthy older people should limit foods and drinks that are rich in sugar, as it can impair dental health and contribute to weight gain if their overall energy intake is too high. However, for people who have a poor appetite, or who have lost weight, sugar-rich foods can be a useful source of calories.

Poor absorption of iron from the gastrointestinal tract and a poor dietary intake, will often lead to anaemia in the older person. Some medicines may also contribute to the development of iron deficiency anaemia, for example, aspirin and ibuprofen, as they can result in bleeding from the stomach. Iron intake can be increased by eating red meat, fortified cereals, and green leafy vegetables.

Calcium loss from bones, which starts at the age of 30 and accelerates considerably in later years, can result in thinning of the bones; this is known as osteoporosis. A person's risk of developing osteoporosis can be reduced by ensuring that calcium rich foods – such as milk, yoghurt, cheese, calcium enriched soya milk and fish containing edible bones – are eaten every day. People who cannot tolerate or dislike these foods may wish to consider taking a calcium supplement. It is also important that older people have enough vitamin D, as this is needed to help reduce calcium loss from the bones. As well as getting vitamin D from dietary sources, the body can synthesise it with exposure to sunlight. Older people may wish to consider taking a vitamin D supplement, as they may not get enough from their diet and the British weather alone.

Older people may also have a low vitamin C intake if they do not consume enough fruit and vegetables. Vitamin C needs to be included in the diet every day, since it cannot be stored in the body. If people find it difficult to eat fruits and vegetables owing to dental problems, fruit juice and soft fruits and vegetables should be included in the diet. Another way to incorporate fruits and vegetables into the diet in a more manageable form is to add them into recipes, such as making fruit desserts or blending them into a homemade soup.

Older people should aim to eat a varied diet, take regular meals and snacks, and drink enough fluid. Sometimes older people cannot eat very much food in a single sitting, so it is important to include nutritious snacks between meals to boost nutrient intake. Good examples include, cheese and biscuits; a fruit yoghurt; two biscuits; a scone; a slice of bread or toast with cheese spread, peanut butter, meat or fish paste; a cereal bar etc.

Some older people may find that their appetite or interest in food lessens to such an extent that they begin to lose weight. If weight loss is noticed, this should be discussed with the person's GP who may decide to refer the individual to a dietitian for assessment and advice. The dietitian may not only encourage nutritious snacks, but also nutritious drinks in their diet, such as full fat milk, malted milk drinks made with full fat milk, or fruit juice. Fortifying foods may be necessary to prevent further weight loss. This is simply the addition of high calorie and high protein ingredients into food to increase the calorie content. For example, cream or dried milk powder can be stirred into porridge and custard, or cheese can be melted on top of savoury dishes. The dietitian will advise which dietary changes are most suitable for the person.

Many older people have poor dentition or poorly fitting dentures. Regular check-ups with the dentist can help to ensure that teeth remain healthy. This will enable older people to enjoy a varied diet that will help maintain their overall health.

HOW CULTURE AND RELIGION AFFECT DIETARY REQUIREMENTS

The Care Quality Commission recommends that service users should have '*a choice for each meal that takes account of their individual preferences and needs, including their religious and cultural requirements*'. (Care Quality Commission, 2010, *Outcome 5: Meeting nutritional needs*)

Culture

The way that we were brought up by our parents, our ethnic background, where we live, our network of friends, and our visits abroad affect our likes and dislikes, our tastes and our eating habits. If a person is used to eating fruits, vegetables, and natural foods, they will find these foods likeable. However, if an individual was brought up eating TV dinners and highly processed foods, then natural foods like vegetables and fruits may not seem so desirable to them.

Cooking techniques have been absorbed into British culture from all over the world, for example, stir-frying. The introduction of masala and balti curries in the 1970s and 1980s has also led to a strong Indian influence in our food. Therefore, it would be wrong to assume, for example, that all older people enjoy traditional British food like steak and kidney pie. Many will have tasted a wide and varied diet during their lifetime and will often enjoy, for example, Indian or Chinese meals. Others will come from minority ethnic groups and their tastes will reflect their own traditional foods.

Religion

As a carer, you need to find out how strictly your service users follow any religious guidelines. While it is essential that you respect their religious beliefs, it is important to realise that one service user might not be as strict as another in applying their religious practices. Some examples of religious dietary guidelines are given below.

Islam

Halal is a Quranic term meaning allowed or lawful. Halal foods and drinks are permitted for consumption by Allah (God) – the supreme law giver. Eating halal food is obligatory for Muslims. Haram, also a Quranic term, means prohibited or unlawful. Haram foods and drinks are absolutely prohibited by Allah, for example, alcohol, animal fat, pork etc. 'Mushbooh' is an Arabic term, which means suspected. If one does not know the halal status of a particular food or drink, that food or drink is doubtful. A practicing Muslim will not consume such foods. In order for meat to be halal, an animal has to be slaughtered in a ritual known as zibah, which states that:

- an animal should not be dead prior to slaughter

- the animal must be fed as normal, and given water prior to slaughter

- an animal must not see another animal being slaughtered

- any flowing blood from the carcass should be completely drained

- slaughtering must not be done in a place where pigs are slaughtered

- a Muslim should perform the slaughter

- the slaughterer and the animal should face Qibla or Mecca.

Judaism

Kosher laws, also known as kashrut, are a guide to food and life for Jewish people. For many Jews, kosher dietary laws are of the highest priority. There are certain foods that are absolutely outlawed, while others can only be consumed in certain combinations or at specific times. The laws:

- restrict the mixing of dairy and meat during meals

- specify the kind of meat that a Jewish person can eat, for example, animals that both chew the cud and have cloven hooves are acceptable

- indicate that fish with gills and scales are kosher, for example, herring, cod, whitefish and salmon, are acceptable; shellfish are not kosher, and scavenger fish may not be

- state that fruits and vegetables are considered kosher.

When shopping in a supermarket, you may see a symbol on some foods that states that a food is 'kosher for Passover'. This means that the factory where the food is produced has been visited by a rabbi who has verified that the food product complies with kosher law. Foods with 'kosher for Passover' symbols can range from seltzer water to matzoh. Matzoh is an unleavened bread consumed during Passover, a Jewish holiday celebrating the freeing of the Jews from slavery in Egypt.

Sikhism

Sikhs do not believe in ritual killing and are told to refrain from eating meat (halal and kosher) killed in such rites. All Sikhs are expected to be active and alert and are therefore required to refrain from alcohol and drugs; not on the grounds of impurity, but for mental and physical fitness. Some Sikhs will not eat beef, others will not eat pork and others will be vegetarian. Because of such varieties and sensitivities, all food served in a gurdwara (Sikh place of worship) is vegetarian.

Hinduism

Food plays an important role in Hindu worship. For example, according to Hindu scripture one should offer all food as a sacrifice to God.
'... All that you do, all that you eat, all that you offer and give away, as well as all austerities that you may perform, should be done as an offering unto Me.' (Bhagavad Gita, 9.27)

The Bhagavad Gita specifies exactly what should be offered:
'If one offers Me with love and devotion a leaf, a flower, a fruit, or water, I will accept it.' (9.26)

Food that is offered to God (prasada) is thought to bestow considerable religious merit, purifying body, mind and spirit. Many Hindus have an altar at home and offer their food before eating. Meat, fish, poultry and eggs are not offered as they are usually considered tamasic (influenced by ignorance). Almost all Hindus avoid eating beef out of respect for the cow. Many Hindus also follow a vegetarian diet. Fasting is common, and Hindus fast as a way to enhance concentration during

meditation or worship, or as purification for the system. Fasting is also sometimes considered a sacrifice. Fasting is dependent on a person's social standing (caste), family, age, gender, and degree of orthodoxy. They can fast by eating 'purer' foods, adopting
a completely vegetarian diet, or by abstaining from favourite foods.

MEDICAL CONDITIONS AFFECTING DIETARY REQUIREMENTS

Many medical conditions require people to follow a special diet for their well-being. There could be serious consequences if the diet is not followed, for example, too much salt could cause fluid retention in kidney patients. The following examples are now discussed:

- coeliac disease

- dementia

- depression

- diabetes

- dysphagia (swallowing difficulties)

- kidney disease.

Coeliac disease

Coeliac disease is a continuing chronic inflammatory condition of the gastrointestinal tract. It is caused by sensitivity to a protein in wheat called gluten. When eaten by someone with coeliac disease, gluten causes inflammatory changes in the lining of the intestine, which impair the gut's ability to absorb nutrients. The condition affects approximately one in 1,000 people in the UK but there is a higher incidence in parts of Ireland. Coeliac disease occurs in other ethnic races, especially those from northern India.

The symptoms of coeliac disease can occur at any age and most people are diagnosed between the ages of 30 and 45 years. Wasting can occur, leading to severe undernourishment or malnutrition. Tiredness and irritability are common. The skin and tongue may show signs of iron deficiency and appear pale. Bones may become brittle, deformed, or may fracture. There is often an increased passage of bulky pale stools with associated abdominal pain and abdominal distension. Women with untreated gluten sensitivity can experience infertility that is restored by withdrawal of gluten from the diet.

Treatment is a strict gluten free diet, for life. Vitamin or mineral supplements may be prescribed to replace any excessive vitamin or mineral loss. Gluten-free foods include all fresh meat, fish, cheese, eggs, milk, fruit and vegetables. However, ordinary bread, pasta, breakfast cereals, biscuits, cakes, pastries, puddings and pies are made from flour, and as they contain gluten, they must be avoided. Gluten is also found in many manufactured and processed foods as wheat flour is commonly used as a processing aid.

Dementia

A person with dementia may have a poor appetite, may forget to eat or that they have already eaten, and are often unaware that they are thirsty. They may therefore become undernourished. A person with dementia may have little interest in food so it is important to include nutritious snacks in between meals to boost their nutrient intake. Good examples include cheese and biscuits; a fruit yoghurt; two biscuits; a scone; a slice of bread or toast with cheese spread, peanut butter, meat or fish paste; a cereal bar etc.

If the person is frail, has lost weight , or has a very small appetite, the nutritional quality of their diet can be improved by using full fat and full sugar versions of food, and by adding high calorie and high protein ingredients, such as milk powder and cheese.

The risk of dehydration can be higher in people with dementia as they are not as sensitive to the feeling of thirst. Dehydration can make a person with dementia drowsy or more confused. Fluid intake doesn't just mean water – it can also include drinks such as tea, coffee, fruit juice and squash. People with dementia who are also at risk of malnutrition should be offered nourishing drinks, such as milky drinks or fruit juice.

Finally, the care worker should be aware that many individuals with dementia may struggle to use cutlery or feed themselves. Adapted cutlery or plate guards can be used, or finger foods can be given. Foods such as fish fingers, potato wedges, cheese cubes and cherry tomatoes can be easily picked up with the hands. Table manners are not important and the care worker should let the person feed themself as much as possible in the way they prefer.

Depression

People who are depressed will often lose interest in everyday activities. They may also feel that they are unable to shop for groceries or prepare food and may lose their appetite. Depression can affect decision-making skills, so planning a daily menu can be extremely difficult. Confidence may also be low and a depressed person may not trust their own ability to cook a meal.

Low blood sugar levels can cause low mood, irritability and fatigue. Therefore, people with depression should be encouraged to eat regularly throughout the day and to not miss meals. They should also be encouraged to avoid sugary foods and drinks as, despite giving a quick rush of energy, they will cause the person to feel tired and low in the long term. It is advisable for people with depression to include foods containing fibre in the diet, such as wholegrain cereals, pulses, fruits and vegetables. Not only can these help to maintain constant blood sugar levels, but they also contain thiamine, a vitamin that may help control mood (Harbottle, 2007).

People with depression should include some protein with every meal to ensure a continuous supply of the amino acid tryptophan to the brain. This is because recent evidence suggests that tryptophan may influence mood. Good sources of protein include meat, fish, eggs, milk, cheese, nuts, beans and lentils. Red meat and fish are also good sources of vitamin B12, another vitamin that may be associated with the control of mood (Harbottle, 2007). When depressed, some individuals may lose interest in food, shopping or cooking, resulting in weight loss. Conversely, others who are depressed may eat more and gain weight. Antidepressants may also affect a person's appetite. Too much weight loss or weight gain can affect the person's mood and should be avoided.

People who are depressed should maintain an adequate fluid intake, as dehydration can affect mod and performance, causing restless or irritable behavior, and loss of concentration. Drinks containing caffeine, such as coffee, tea and some fizzy drinks, may be used to boost energy levels but in large quantities they may cause anxiety, sleep problems and increase the symptoms of depression. Caffeine can also increase the risk of developing dehydration as it is a mild diuretic, so intake should be limited to no more than three to four cups of coffee or equivalent per day. Water, fruit juices or decaffeinated drinks can be taken instead.

Alcohol depresses brain activity and can influence mood. It is also a toxin that has to be deactivated by the liver, which uses several essential vitamins. Certain vitamin deficiencies are common in heavy drinkers and can cause low mood, irritability or aggressive behaviour. People with depression should avoid consuming alcohol.

Exercise leads to the release of endorphins – feel-good chemicals that help us to relax and feel happy. Exercise is particularly important for people with depression as it can also give some structure to the day.

For further information on healthy eating and depression see Healthy Eating and Depression (Mental Health Foundation, 2007) available online at: www.mentalhealth.org.uk/content/assets/PDF/publications/healthy_eating_depression.pdf

Diabetes

People with diabetes have abnormally high levels of glucose in their blood. There are two types of diabetes: type 1 and type 2.

- **Type 1** is more likely to be present in younger people. It develops when the cells in the pancreas that produce insulin are destroyed. Insulin is a hormone that is needed to regulate levels of glucose in the blood. This type of diabetes is treated with insulin injections.

- **Type 2** diabetes is usually diagnosed in older people. It is treated with diet and exercise, although some people with type 2 diabetes may need medication and may sometimes require insulin too.

People with diabetes can live an active, normal and healthy life. However, poorly controlled diabetes can lead to complications such as heart disease, kidney disease, blindness and nerve and circulatory problems, which may result in the amputation of limbs. To prevent any long-term complications it is extremely important to control blood sugar levels and blood pressure for both types of diabetes.

People are more likely to develop type 2 diabetes if they:

■ have a relative with diabetes

■ are overweight

■ are aged over 40

■ are of Asian or African-Caribbean origin

■ have had diabetes during pregnancy.

People with diabetes should try to watch their weight and eat a diet that:

■ is low in saturated fat

■ is low in sugar

■ is low in salt

■ contains at least five portions of fruit or vegetables a day

■ is high in wholegrain, starchy carbohydrate foods, such as wholegrain bread, chapattis, rice, and pasta.

People with diabetes should try to eat only small amounts of foods that are high in sugar or fat, or both. They can eat cakes and biscuits occasionally but only as part of a balanced diet.

Low blood sugar (hypoglycaemia) can occur when diabetes is treated with insulin or certain tablets (sulphonylureas). If the person with diabetes has hypoglycaemia they may sometimes need to increase their blood sugar level quickly. This can be done with a sugary drink or some glucose tablets, followed by a starchy snack, such as a sandwich.

Dysphagia

Dysphagia is a difficulty swallowing or a disturbance in the normal movement of food from the mouth to the stomach. Dysphagia can lead to choking and aspiration of food into the lungs, causing chest infections and pneumonia. It can also cause inadequate nutrition and weight loss. Possible causes of dysphagia include stroke, head and neck injury, Parkinson's disease and multiple sclerosis. There are two main types:

■ difficulty emptying food from the back of the mouth into the oesophagus

■ difficulty passing food along the oesophagus into the stomach.

A person with dysphagia will commonly cough when eating, drool or pocket food in the cheeks. If a difficulty with swallowing is suspected, a speech and language therapist (SLT) should be consulted to evaluate the person's swallowing ability. If swallowing ability is compromised the SLT may be able to teach swallowing techniques to improve the quality of the swallow. The SLT may also recommend that fluids are thickened and that the texture of food is modified to help make swallowing easier and to help prevent choking.

It is important to include a wide variety of foods and nutrients in the diet. For example, if puréed food is advised by the SLT, it is vital to provide a balanced and nutritious diet. Many foods can be puréed to provide balanced meals and snacks. Further advice about this can be obtained from a dietitian.

In the case of severe swallowing difficulties, it may be unsafe for the person to take food and fluid orally, resulting in the need for feeding via a tube. This may be via a nasogastric tube, which is passed through the nose and into the stomach, or via a gastrostomy tube, which is passed directly through the stomach wall. Nasogastric tubes are usually a short-term method of feeding, whereas gastrostomy tubes are used in the long term. You may hear of gastrostomy tubes being referred to as PEGs; this stands for percutaneous endoscopic gastrostomy, which describes how the gastrostomy tube is passed – through the stomach wall with the aid of an endsoscope (see **Figures 1 and 2**).

Figure 1: PEG feeding tube

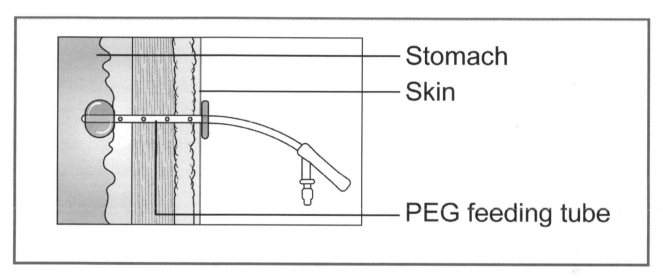

Taken from CancerHelp UK (2010a), the patient website of Cancer Research UK www.cancerhelp.org.uk

Figure 2: Feeding via a PEG tube

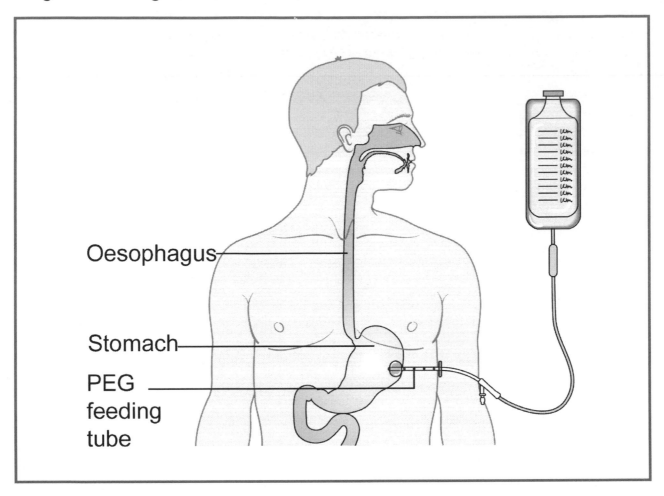

Oesophagus

Stomach

PEG feeding tube

Taken from CancerHelp UK (2010b), the patient website of Cancer Research UK www.cancerhelp.org.uk

Once the feeding tube has been placed and it is confirmed that it is in the correct position, feed, fluid and medications can be administered. A syringe will be used to give medications and may also be used to provide feed and fluid. Many people use a feeding pump however, which can be set up to gradually administer a bag of feed over a number of hours (see **Figure 2**). The dietitian will provide a feeding regimen that clearly states the feed to be used and the speed and duration of feeding that the feeding pump should be set to.

It is important that both the gastrostomy tube and site are well cared for to prevent complications such as infections. The gastrostomy tube should be flushed well with water every day, especially after medications, as these can block the tube. The gastrostomy site should be kept clean. Guidance for the correct cleaning of the gastrostomy site will be provided by the hospital where the gastrostomy was placed, and must be followed. Individuals who receive PEG feeds are at risk of regurgitation or reflux of the feed, which can cause choking, or which can be aspirated into the lungs and cause a chest infection. Therefore, individuals who are PEG fed are usually sat upright at an angle of at least 45 degrees while the feed is in progress, and they should remain in this position for at least 30 minutes after the feed has been discontinued.

It is important to ensure that the individual's mouth is cared for and the mucous membranes remain moist in order to avoid infections such as thrush. A soft toothbrush should be used to cleanse the teeth and gums, and Vaseline or lip salve can be applied to prevent cracking of the lips and corners of the mouth. Some individuals may be able to sip fluids or suck ice lollies or ice cubes, if the SLT advises that this is safe. Artificial saliva can be prescribed by the GP and applied to the tongue if required.

Kidney disease

The kidneys are responsible for removing toxins from our blood and disposing of them through the urine. If the kidneys are not working correctly, the body retains fluid, which will begin to build up in lungs, the heart, and the abdominal cavity. People with kidney failure struggle to get rid of body fluids and any additional salt (sodium) retained in their body can cause problems. Physicians will test the person's urine and blood to assess the level of renal function, which is then graded. Medication may be prescribed to control the symptoms and progress of the person's kidney disease. Dietary advice may be required to help control the levels of certain minerals in the blood.

Dietary advice is particularly important when dialysis begins, but will depend on an individual's blood levels and the type of dialysis, for example, whether it is the kind carried out at home (peritoneal dialysis) or at hospital (haemodialysis).

Sodium should be restricted for every renal patient and they should follow a no added salt diet. This means reducing the amount of salt added to cooking, not adding salt to meals and reducing high salt foods. Foods which are high in salt include: processed meat products, such as ham, sausage, bacon, corned beef; hard cheeses; fast foods; pickles; soy sauce and Chinese or oriental foods. Sodium is also present in commercially prepared foods. Canned fish or vegetables in spring water or oils are preferable to those in brine.

Fluids may also need to be restricted for people with kidney disease. This will be advised by a GP and dietitian. For dialysis patients the recommended fluid intake is usually 500ml plus the previous day's urine output. Gravies and custards may need to be included in this allowance in some cases.

In addition, potassium intake may need to be controlled. The highest amounts of potassium are found in bananas, baked beans, mushrooms, nuts, avocados, potatoes (if not boiled), butternut squash, apricots, mango and dried fruits. Low potassium foods include blackberries, grapes, tangerines, canned pears and plums, green or waxed beans, corn, cauliflower, broccoli, carrots and cucumbers. Phosphate in foods may also need to be avoided. Dairy products, nuts, tinned fish, prawns, crab and organ meats all contain phosphate. Cola is also high in phosphate. High phosphate foods are usually also high in protein, therefore the dietitian will advise on the restrictions if they are necessary, and the quantities allowed.

THE PREPARATION AND PRESENTATION OF FOOD AND DRINK

Preparation of food

It is really important when preparing and serving food to frail older people that strict hygiene rules are adhered to in order to prevent food poisoning. Good personal hygiene is key to good food hygiene, as food can become contaminated by touch. You should always wash your hands, and the hands of your service users, thoroughly before handling food. In addition, you should wash your hands after visiting the toilet, smoking, or after completing any personal care, as your hands will have become contaminated during these activities. You should wear a plastic apron or clean tabard over your uniform to ensure that germs are not transported from your clothes to any food you are handling.

The attractiveness of food

Food and drink should be *'presented in an appetising way to encourage enjoyment'* (Care Quality Commission, 2010). In order to encourage frail older people to eat, food must be attractively presented. For example, serving chicken with mashed potato and cauliflower provides a balanced meal but will be visually unappealing as all the components are a similar colour. The addition of different coloured vegetables can make such a meal more tempting. Portion size is also important as a very full plate could look overwhelming to an individual with a poor appetite.

Food consistency

The consistency of food relates to how soft or hard the food is. The texture of food is sensed by the tongue and palate. It could be crispy, crunchy or slimy in texture and these different sensations can often be used to stimulate a service user's appetite. Some individuals may dislike certain textures; however, it is very important to provide clients with the correct texture of food and fluid as advised by the SLT. It is also very important that the care worker pays attention to the service user's oral hygiene, as some foods, for example, pips from fruit, can get trapped under dentures, causing irritation.

As discussed previously, people with swallowing difficulties may need the texture of their food modified, for example, food could be puréed. Food thickeners may be added to liquids on advice from an SLT, to assist individuals who have swallowing difficulties. A soft diet includes foods that are easily chewed, such as minced beef or rice pudding.

The temperature of food

Meals should be served at an appropriate temperature. Hot meals should be given to individuals before they become cold, as this could cause the service user to lose interest in their food. If the individual requires assistance with feeding, staff should help them straight away rather than waiting until the food gets cold. If the service user is a slow eater, the food may need to be kept warm or to be reheated, but food should only be reheated once. There is a risk of receiving burns from food that is served too hot, for example, hot drinks or foods that have been reheated in the microwave. Ensuring that food is served at the correct temperature will also help to avoid food poisoning.

Variety

A varied and diverse diet is required to ensure that meals are nutritionally balanced. The intake of some individuals who eat a restricted diet may be lacking in essential vitamins. If this is the case, the dietitian can offer dietary advice.

Supplementary foods

Individuals who are malnourished or who are at risk of malnutrition should be referred to a dietitian who can assess their diet and provide advice on how to increase its nutritional value. This can be achieved through dietary changes such as snacks, nourishing drinks and food fortification. Some individuals may also require nutritional supplements on prescription. A GP or dietitian can advise whether these are indicated.

Reconstitution and moulding of food

As discussed earlier in the chapter, some individuals who have difficulty with swallowing may need to have their food puréed. The problem is that once the texture of the food has changed it can often look unappetising. Puréed food can be made to look more attractive by puréeing the foods separately and serving these in separate sections on the plate. Different coloured foods should be used to make the meal look more appealing. Piping puréed food onto the plate or the use of food moulds can also improve its appearance.

Preparation of food by service users

The Care Quality Commission's *Guidance about Compliance: Essential standards of quality and safety* (2010) states '*people who use services should be actively supported to plan and prepare their own meals, where this is safe and they are able to do so.*' There is, of course, health and safety legislation that prevents service users from using a care home's main kitchen. However, the Care Quality Commission (CQC) recommends that care homes provide kitchenettes for individuals to use. These could, for example, contain a small toaster or microwave with grill, which service users can use to make their own drinks or prepare sandwiches or small snacks such as cheese on toast. In addition, the CQC recommends that care homes organise cooking activities for service users, for example, baking cookies or scones that can be served with afternoon tea.

CREATING AN APPROPRIATE ENVIRONMENT

Eating and drinking aids

'*People who use services can be confident that staff will support them to meet their eating and drinking needs with sensitivity and respect for their dignity and ability. They are enabled to eat their food and drink as independently as possible. All assistance necessary is provided to ensure they actually eat and drink, where they want to but are unable to do so independently. They have supportive equipment available to them that allows them to eat and drink independently, wherever needed.'* (Care Quality Commission, 2010, *Outcome 5: Meeting nutritional needs*)

It is important that service users remain independent with eating and drinking for as long as possible, as this will help to maintain their self-esteem. There are a number of online shops that sell various aids to assist people with eating and drinking, some examples are listed below.

■ Essential Aids (www.essentialaids.com)

■ Mobility World (www.mobilityworld.co.uk)

■ The Disabled Shop (www.thedisabledshop.com)

■ The Stroke Shop (www.strokeshop.org.uk)

■ Welcome Mobility (www.welcomemobility.co.uk)

For example, this elastic strap with hook and loop closure can be used with utensils that may have a built-up handle. It may be useful for service users with limited hand function.

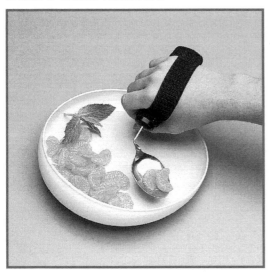

This lightweight plastic cup is for people with limited strength or poor co-ordination.

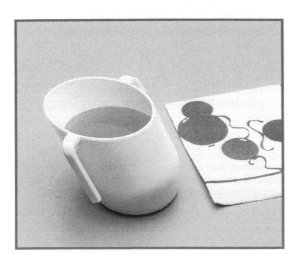

The curved rim on this bowl will guide food onto a spoon while the slip-resistant base helps keep the bowl firmly in place.

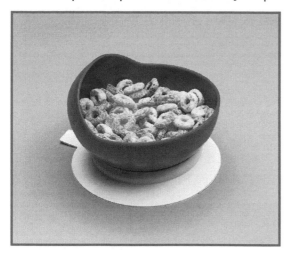

These spoons are ideal for people with limited co-ordination. The coated spoons have built-up handles that are easy to hold even when wet. The coating also protects teeth and lips. These are ideal for clients with spasticity or limited hand control.

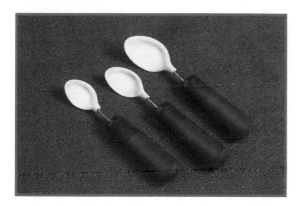

This food guard has a snug fit, which means that the food guard stays on the plate securely when food is scooped up against it – so that food doesn't slip off the plate. Tapered ends prevent the food guard from interfering with utensils.

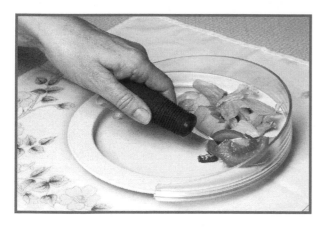

Photographs courtesy of The Disabled Shop: www.thedisabledshop.com

Choice of food

Care Quality Commission *Guidance about Compliance: Essential standards of quality and safety. Outcome 5 – Meeting nutritional needs* (2010) states that:

'[service users should] … have accessible information about meals and the arrangements for mealtimes and have a choice for each meal that takes account of their individual preferences and needs, including their religious and cultural requirements'.

This indicates that care homes must provide a menu that is changed regularly. This should offer a choice of meals in written or other formats, for example, Braille, to suit the capacities of all service users. This must be given to and read or explained to service users.

Environment

When assisting frail older people to eat and drink, you should ensure that:

- meals are served in a quiet place so that the person can focus on eating, for example, the television or radio should be turned off

- the table setting is kept simple, for example, remove flowers, centre pieces and condiments, and only use the utensils needed for the meal

- the person can distinguish food from their plate or bowl, for example, avoid highly patterned dishes, tablecloths and placemats

- the food is at the correct temperature as the service user might not be able to tell if food or beverages are too hot to eat or drink

- the service user is given plenty of time to eat

- the independence of the service user is encouraged by making the most of their abilities, for example, the person could eat from a bowl instead of a plate, or with a spoon instead of a fork.

End of chapter quiz

1. List six essential nutrients for a healthy diet.

2. Outline the eight healthy eating tips recommended by the NHS Choices Live Well website.

3. Why is iron needed in the body?

4. Give three risk factors for premature death in adults.

5. How might these risk factors be limited through diet?

6. How might you alter the diet for an older person to compensate for weight loss?

7. What is osteoporosis?

8. How might you increase dietary intake of calcium?

9. What are the risks associated with PEG feeding?

10. What position should a person receiving a PEG feed be nursed in?

✍ My continuing professional development (CPD) log

Name of care worker ....

Name of manager/supervisor ....

Name of employer ....

Start date for training...

Expected date of completion ....

This is to confirm that .... [*name of care worker*] has satisfactorily completed...................... [*insert number*] of hours of study, and has achieved all of the following learning points:

- The factors that may affect the dietary requirements of individuals, for example, age, culture, religion, medical conditions, availability of food etc

- The importance of appropriate preparation and presentation of food and drink, for example, attractiveness, consistency, temperature, variety etc

- The importance of creating an appropriate environment in which to eat and drink, for example, use of eating aids, choice of menu, environment etc

Comments from care worker or supervisor, for example, outcomes of key learning activities or results of quiz.

Signed (care worker): .... Date:..............................

Signed (supervisor): .... Date:..............................

Chapter two

Roles and boundaries

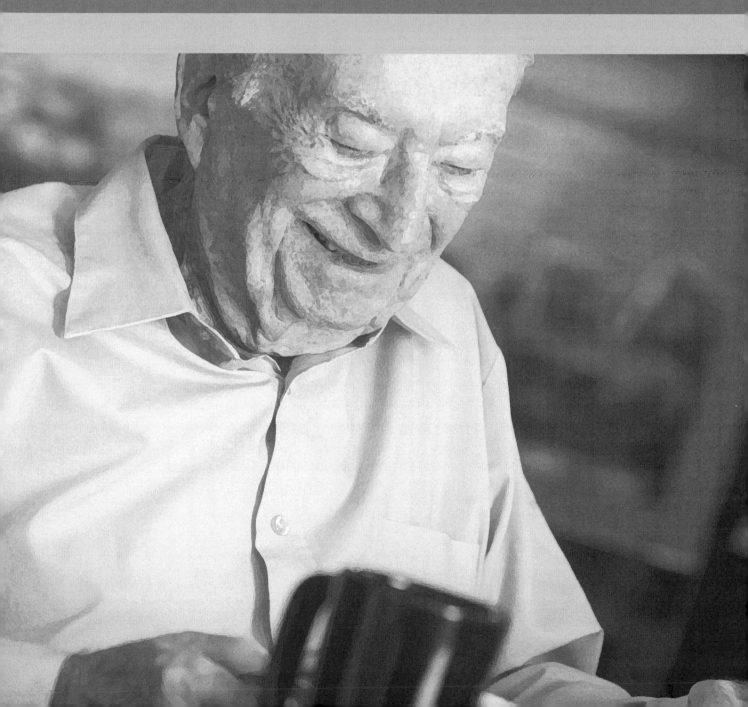

Chapter two

Roles and boundaries

☺ Key learning activity

This activity will provide you with the key background information before you read **Chapter two**. Make a note of your answers and discuss these with a colleague or your supervisor before you start your reading.

Go to www.nhs.uk/Tools/Pages/Healthyweightcalculator.aspx

Q1. How would you define the term body mass index (BMI)?

Q2. Calculate your own BMI using the tool provided on the website.

Go to www.nhs.uk/conditions/Food-poisoning/Pages/Introduction.aspx

Q3. What are the causes of food poisoning?

Q4. What are the signs and symptoms of food poisoning?

Q5. How can food poisoning be prevented?

AIMS OF THE CHAPTER

At the end of this chapter, the reader will have considered the role, responsibilities and boundaries of the care worker in relation to:

- workplace policies and procedures that may influence the assessment of dietary need, for example, nutritional screening, person-centred approaches to care etc

- the monitoring of individual dietary therapies, for example, documentation and record keeping, observing and reporting, seeking guidance and advice etc

- the handling and serving of food to service users, for example, food hygiene, personal hygiene assisting with eating etc

- personnel who are involved in the nutrition and well-being of service users, for example, kitchen staff, speech and language therapist, dietitian etc.

This chapter covers the underpinning knowledge for the following Level 2 mandatory and optional units in food safety and nutrition (the number following each relates to a learning outcome):

- HSC 2014:4

- HSC 2014:5

- HSC 2029:1

- HSC2029:2

- HSC 2029:3

- FSN 201:3

- FSN 201:6

- FSN 301:4

- FSN 301:5

- FSN 301:7

- FSN 301:8

WORKPLACE POLICIES AND PROCEDURES

Nutritional screening

It is estimated that over 3 million people in Britain are malnourished (undernourished). Malnutrition has a number of adverse effects on health, including increased risk of infections and delayed recovery from illness. It is therefore extremely costly to the NHS. The British Association for Parenteral and Enteral Nutrition (BAPEN) suggests that in the UK approximately £13 billion is spent each year as a result of malnutrition (BAPEN, 2010).

The Age UK (formerly Age Concern) report *Still Hungry to be Heard* (2010) highlights the poor nutritional state of vulnerable and older people receiving institutional care. According to the report, the number of people leaving hospital who are malnourished is increasing: 157,175 people left hospital malnourished in 2007/8; this rose to 185,446 in 2008/9.

Age UK states that older malnourished individuals are more likely to stay in hospital longer and are three times more likely to develop complications from surgery. In short, Age UK states that undernourished individuals receiving institutional care have a higher mortality rate than those who are well fed.

Age UK (2010), the National Institute for Health and Clinical Excellence (2006) and BAPEN (undated) each consider that nutritional screening of people at risk of malnutrition, such as older people being admitted to institutional care, is of vital importance. In order to identify individuals who are at risk of malnutrition, a screening tool, such as the Malnutrition Universal Screening Tool (MUST), should be used. MUST assesses body mass index, unintentional weight loss and the presence of acute illness resulting in negligible or no dietary intake, to determine whether the individual is at low, medium or high risk of malnutrition.

☺ Activity: Calculate your own BMI

Body mass index (BMI) is generally used to assess whether an adult's weight is healthy, or if they are under or overweight.

To calculate

Body mass index is calculated by dividing weight in kilograms by height in metres squared. For example, a person weighing 80 kilograms and standing 1.6 metres tall would have a BMI of 31:

- 80 ÷ (1.6 x 1.6) = 80 ÷ 2.56 = 31.25

What does the score mean?

- BMI less than 20: Underweight

- BMI 20–24.9: Ideal

- BMI 25–29.9: Overweight

- BMI greater than 30: Obese

The National Institute for Health and Clinical Excellence (2006) states that anyone who has a BMI of less than 18.5, who has lost more than 10% body weight unintentionally in three to six months, or who has a BMI of less than 20 and has lost five to 10% body weight unintentionally in three to six months, is likely to be malnourished.

What is your BMI? Use the above formula to calculate it.

MUST ASSESSMENT TOOL

BAPEN recommends that the Malnutrition Universal Screening Tool (MUST) should be used. MUST is a five-step screening tool developed by BAPEN, which generates a score to identify adults who are malnourished or at risk of malnutrition. It also provides guidelines that can be used to develop a nutritional care plan. The steps of the MUST tool are as follows.

Step 1

A person's height and weight are measured to get a BMI score. If the BMI is less than 18.5 this gives a score of 2. If the BMI is 18.5 to 20 this gives a score of 1. If the BMI is greater than 20 this gives a score of 0.

Step 2

If the weight loss is greater than 10% this gives a score of 2. If the weight loss is between five per cent and 10%, this gives a score of 1. If it is less than five per cent this gives a score of 0.

Step 3

The effect of acute disease is scored. If the service user is acutely ill and there has been, or is likely to be, no nutritional intake for more than five days, this gives a score of 2. Otherwise the score is 0.

Step 4

Add the scores from steps 1, 2 and 3 together to obtain an overall score for risk of malnutrition. A total score of:

- 0 = low risk

- 1 = medium risk

- 2 or more = high risk.

Step 5

Develop a care plan in accordance with your local nutrition policy or guidelines. Contact your local dietetic department for advice if required. Some example care plans follow.

- **Score 0 = low risk.** Provide routine care. Rescreen the individual on an annual basis or sooner if concern arises.

- **Score 1 = medium risk.** Keep food charts for three days to assess the individual's dietary intake. Offer nourishing snacks and nourishing drinks. Rescreen the person monthly.

- **Score of more than 2 = high risk.** Keep food charts for three days to assess the individual's dietary intake. Offer nourishing snacks and nourishing drinks. Fortify meals and drinks with high calorie and high protein ingredients. Discuss the individual's situation with the GP and consider referral to a dietitian. Weigh the person weekly and rescreen them monthly.

PERSON-CENTRED APPROACHES

Fundamental to the person-centred approach is the need to recognise a person's:

- culture

- individuality

- feelings

- need for privacy

- need for respect.

Culture

When caring for someone it is important that staff understand a person's cultural or religious background and any rules or customs that may apply. This will include the need to:

- use respectful forms of address, for example, *'Would you like some potatoes Mr Smith?'* rather than *'Would you like some potatoes, luv?'*

- understand forms of touch or gesture that are considered to be disrespectful

- establish religious observances, such as fasting

- identify how and what the person prefers to eat, for example, *'Here is the menu for tomorrow Mr Smith, would you prefer the roast dinner or the salad?'*

Individuality

An individual's sense of who they are is closely connected to the name they are called. Therefore, it is important that you address the person in a way that the person recognises and prefers. For example, some people may be happy to be called by their first name or nickname, while others may prefer to be addressed as Mr or Mrs. Many vulnerable people have a fragile sense of self-worth, therefore it is important that they are treated with courtesy. Care staff should:

- be kind and reassure the person without talking down to them

- never talk over the person's head as if they are not there, for example, *'Mrs Smith wants soup, don't you dear'*

- include the person in conversations

- avoid criticising or making the person feel small, for example, *'Mrs Smith you haven't eaten a thing, you'll get me into trouble if you don't clear your plate'*

- try to imagine how they would like to be spoken to if they were in the same position

- listen carefully to the person, even if they don't seem to be making much sense, as they are trying to communicate how they feel.

Feelings

A vulnerable person is likely, at times, to be sad or upset and they may want to talk about any worries or concerns they have. It is important that care staff:

- make time to offer support, for example, *'I'll sit down and help you. Don't worry, there is plenty of time, so please don't rush your meal'*

- listen and show the person that they are there for them

- recognise how the person is feeling; they may be able to judge this from the person's expression and/or body language, for example, *'I can see by your face that you don't like the soup Mrs Smith. Is that correct?'*

- always explain what they are doing, and why, for example, *'You have lost quite a bit of weight recently, so the dietitian has come to talk with you about your diet. Is this OK Mrs Smith?'*

- phrase questions carefully so that they only need a 'yes' or 'no' answer, as too much choice can often add to the person's confusion, for example, *'Mrs Smith, would you like vegetable soup to start with?'* rather than *'Would you like the soup, the salad or the pâté to start with Mrs Smith?'*

- give the person every opportunity to make their own choices by informing and consulting with the person about matters that concern them, for example, *'Mrs Smith, your husband tells me that you don't eat red meat, what would you prefer instead?'*.

Privacy

The person's right to privacy must be respected, for example, care staff should always knock on a person's bedroom door before entering. If the person requires personal and intimate care, such as assistance with eating and drinking, this must be done sensitively, and adequate time and an appropriate environment must be arranged.

Respect

When an older person finds that their mental abilities are declining, they often feel vulnerable and in need of reassurance and support. Service users need to feel respected and valued. In order to do this carers need to:

- do things with the person, rather than for them, to help them retain their independence, for example, *'I'm going to sit and have a cup of tea with you while you have your drink Mrs Smith, is that OK?'*

- avoid situations in which the person is likely to fail, as this can be humiliating, for example, ensure that a plate guard is in place to avoid spillage of food onto the table (see **Chapter one**)

- look for tasks and activities that the individual can still manage and enjoy, for example, helping to prepare meals, setting the table or pouring a glass of wine to drink with their meal

- break activities down into small steps so that the person feels a sense of achievement, even if they can only manage part of a task

- let individuals do things at their own pace and in their own way, for example, let them have plenty of time to eat their meal or allow them to eat their pudding first, if they wish

- give plenty of praise and encouragement.

Many of your service users will need help with eating and drinking. They might not be physically capable of feeding themselves because of a disability. They might be confused or disorientated and might not recognise the need to eat or drink. They might have temporarily lost their appetite because of the effects of an acute illness, ill-fitting dentures or medication.

Age UK (formerly Age Concern) and the Royal College of Nursing (2007a) provide the following tips for assisting the individual to eat and drink.

1. Adequately prepare individuals for their meals.

An individual is more likely to feel like eating if they are clean, comfortable and relaxed before each meal arrives. Care workers can ensure this by:

- assisting individuals to go to the toilet and ensuring their hands are washed

- brushing teeth, freshening the mouth and ensuring that dentures are fitted

- putting hearing aids in and spectacles back on

- sitting the person upright in bed or in a chair

- clearing tables of any clutter to minimise distractions

- making sure there are no unpleasant sights, smells or sounds.

2. Set up meal trays or tables correctly.

It is important to support older people to eat by themselves, and to allow plenty of time for this. You can help by making sure food is within reach and is easy to handle by:

- adjusting tables to the right height

- removing wrappers and lids

- cutting up food into manageable pieces

- buttering bread and peeling fruit

- putting straws in drinks (not advised for people with dysphagia)

- providing special cutlery (see **Chapter one**).

3. Provide appropriate help with eating.

Some individuals will require assistance to eat and drink. Care workers should:

- sit in front of them and make eye contact

- give small amounts at a time and pause between each mouthful

- offer a drink at regular intervals

- mix food with gravy or sauces to make it easier for people to chew and swallow the food (if their diet allows)

- allow plenty of time.

4. Offer encouragement.

When an individual is feeling ill, they are more likely to refuse food. It is important that they try and eat something – even if it's just a little. Care workers can help by:

- being pleasant and friendly

- speaking positively about the food

- serving less food more often

- encouraging nutritionally dense snacks between meals (see **Chapter one**).

5. Talk with the service user and observe them.

Through conversation and observation, the care worker can identify any problems the person may have with:

- eating and drinking, for example, swallowing

- the food, for example, is it cold? Does it taste and look good?

Any concerns should be reported to the care worker's supervisor.

☺ Activity: Assisting an individual to eat and drink

Think about somebody you support and the particular assistance they need in order to be able to eat and drink. In the table below identify specific ways that you would support the individual to eat and drink, according to the different types of help. You might want to discuss this with a colleague before completing the following table.

Assisting an individual to eat and drink

Type of help	Specific support you would provide
Preparing the person	
Setting up the meal tray/table	
Providing help while the person eats	
Offering encouragement	
Talking to and observing the person	

MONITORING THE DIET OF VULNERABLE INDIVIDUALS

Monitoring daily progress

Age UK and The Royal College of Nursing (2007b) offer the following advice when monitoring the dietary habits of older people who are receiving institutional care ie. care workers should check for, record and report:

- any significant weight loss (over half a stone in the last three to six months)
- any recent loss of appetite
- any loose fitting clothes
- signs of recurrent infections
- any difficulty recovering from illness
- any loss of ability to keep warm
- constipation or diarrhoea
- pressure sores
- any ill-fitting dentures
- swollen or bleeding gums
- a sore mouth or tongue
- difficulties chewing or swallowing
- tooth decay.

If the care worker notices any of these signs they must discuss it with their supervisor and record it in the service user's care plan.

Principles of good record keeping

Care plans, nutritional screening, weight charts, dietary and fluid intake charts are required as legal records of care, and the keeping of certain confidential notes and records relating to individual service users are an essential part of the communication and day-to-day running of a care home.

Examples of recording charts

LAWNS NURSING HOME

24-hour fluid chart

Name: Date of birth:

Date:

Time	Fluid	Amount	Urine	Vomit	Aspirate (PEG)	Comments
0800	Tea	180	300			MSU taken
0900	Juice	50				Sips only
1000	Coffee	180				
1200	Soup	200				
Total 24 hrs						

MUST NUTRITION CARE PLAN

Medium risk (MUST score 1)

Resident's name......Mrs X.......................... Room.........xx.............................

Date care plan started...25/3/2011...

Action	Date and initials				
	25/3/2011	25/04/2011			
Record weight and all MUST scores in resident's notes using MUST recording sheet.	ABC	ABC			
Record all food eaten for three days. File completed food charts in resident's notes.	ABC	ABC			
Provide fortified food and fluids. Ensure that kitchen staff are fortifying food. Encourage high calorie snacks between meals and high calorie drinks.	ABC	ABC			
Every month (or earlier if you are concerned) screen resident again using MUST.		ABC			

Action	Date and initials				
	25/3/2011	25/04/2011			
Every month review this care plan. If resident's MUST risk changes, change the care plan.		ABC			
Record progress with this care plan in the notes section overleaf.	ABC	ABC			

Tick any special requirements that apply:

Resident requires help with choosing meals and snacks ☑

Resident requires help with feeding and drinking ☑

Resident requires modified tableware ☐

Resident requires modified texture: Soft ☑

(advised by speech and language therapist owing   Puréed ☐

to difficulty swallowing)   Thickened fluids ☐

Resident's food preferences are:...Puddings...Eggs...

....

....

....

Date	Notes	Initials
25/3/11	Spoken with kitchen – they are fortifying all food. Food charts show good intake at breakfast and likes puddings, therefore encourage these.	ABC
25/4/11	Weight stable now. Having cooked breakfast sometimes and often manages two puddings.	ABC

© Peterborough Community Services Nutrition and Dietetic Department, January 2011

The NHS Confidentiality Code of Practice (DH, 2003) suggests the following guidelines for care records.

1. Records must be factual, consistent and accurate ie. they should be:

■ written as soon as possible after an event has occurred, providing current information on the care and condition of the service user

■ written clearly, legibly and in such a manner that they cannot be erased

- written in such a manner that any alterations or additions are dated, timed and signed so that the original entry can still be read clearly

- accurately dated, timed and signed or otherwise identified, with the name of the author being printed alongside the first entry

- readable on any photocopies ie. care records should be written in black ink

- written, wherever applicable, with the involvement of the service user

- clear, unambiguous, (preferably concise) and written in terms that the service user can understand.

2. Records must be relevant and useful ie. they should:

- identify problems that have arisen and the action taken to rectify them

- provide evidence of the care planned, the decisions made, the care delivered and the information shared

- provide evidence of actions agreed with the service user (including consent to care and/or consent to disclose information).

3. Care records should not include:

- unnecessary abbreviations or jargon

- meaningless phrases, irrelevant speculation or offensive subjective statements

- irrelevant personal opinions regarding the service user.

Legislation and record keeping

The rules governing the recording and use of service user information are set out by *The Caldicott Report* (DH, 1995). The key requirements of this report are that the care worker must:

- justify a purpose for recording and using service user information

- only record and use information when it is absolutely necessary

- use only the minimum information required

- only access information on a strict 'need to know' basis

- be aware of their responsibilities concerning the recording and use of service user information

- understand and comply with the law, for example, the Data Protection Act (1998) (DPA).

Care Quality Commission *Guidance about Compliance: Essential standards of quality and safety. Outcome 1 - Respecting and involving people who use services* (2010) states that: '*People who use services:*

- *can express their views, so far as they are able to do so, and are involved in making decisions about their care, treatment and support*

- *have their privacy, dignity and independence respected*

- *have their views and experiences taken into account in the way the service is provided and delivered.'*

This can be done in the case of record keeping by encouraging staff to involve the service user whenever records are being written. If this is done then not only can the service user be more actively involved in their own care, but the need for the recording can be explained and understood. By developing an atmosphere of 'working together' with the service user, anxieties will be greatly reduced.

The Care Quality Commission's *Guidance about Compliance: Essential standards of quality and safety* (2010) *Outcome 21* relates to the degree to which service users' rights and best interests are safeguarded by a home's record keeping policies and procedures. Specific standards include the following.

- *'The service has clear procedures that are followed in practice, monitored and reviewed, to ensure personalised records and medical records are kept and maintained for each person who uses the service.'*

- *'Records about people who use services are used to plan appropriate care, treatment and support to ensure their rights and best interests are protected and their needs are met.'*

- *'Records are securely stored and transferred internally between departments and externally to other organisations, when required.'*

The Data Protection Act (1998)

The Data Protection Act (1998) (DPA) sets standards governing the storage and processing of personal data held in manual records and on computers. The act works in two ways – giving individuals (data subjects) certain rights, while requiring those who record and use personal information (data controllers) to be open about their use of that information and to follow sound and proper practices (the data protection principles). All residential or nursing care homes that hold manual or computerised service user or employee records are covered by the DPA. According to the DPA, there are eight main principles under which personal data should be kept and collected. Personal data should:

- be obtained fairly and lawfully

- be held for specified and lawful purposes

- be processed in accordance with the person's rights under the DPA

- be adequate, relevant and not excessive in relation to that purpose

- be kept accurate and up-to-date

- not be kept for longer than is necessary for the given purpose

- be subject to appropriate safeguards against unauthorised use, loss or damage.

One of the most important aspects of the DPA is that personal data may be processed only if the service user has given their consent. All files kept about residents or staff should be confidential and, according to the DPA, service users should know what records are being kept about them and why they are being kept.

Service users should also be given access to what is said about them in any personal records maintained by the home and information should be withheld only in exceptional circumstances. All data, particularly sensitive or confidential data, must be stored securely. Manual records such as personnel files and resident care files should be kept in locked filing cabinets, preferably in an office that is locked when unattended. Care must be taken when working on confidential files to make sure that they are put away securely and not left out on a desk where people could walk by and see them. Care records will ensure that service user information will remain confidential.

FOOD HANDLING

In order for you to understand the importance of correct food handling it is appropriate for you to review:

1. how infection is spread

2. who is most at risk of infection

3. what measures you can take to reduce the risk of infection.

1. How infection is spread

Infectious diseases are caused by:

- bacteria, (for example, food poisoning)

- viruses, (for example, influenza)

- fungi, (for example, thrush).

These can be spread by:
- direct contact – being touched by an infectious person (for example, scabies)

- indirect contact – touching materials an infected person has used (for example, impetigo)

- inhalation – breathing in infected droplets from a cough or sneeze (for example, influenza)

- ingestion – from contaminated food (for example, *Salmonella* food poisoning)

- injection – from a needle stick injury (for example, HIV or hepatitis B).

2. Who is most at risk of infection?

The vulnerable adult is often at risk from infectious or communicable diseases because their immunity to micro-organisms such as bacteria and viruses may be low. This might be because of the medicines they are taking, or their nutritional state might be poor.

3. Measures you can take to reduce the risk of infection

Infection control, or the ways in which the spread of infection might be reduced is an important part of a care worker's job. One of the most important measures you can take to prevent the spread of any infection is a correct hand washing technique, particularly before you:

- handle food
- give out any medicines
- give emergency first aid
- handle any wounds.

You should also wash your hands after you:
- use the toilet
- assist others to use the toilet
- cough, sneeze or use a handkerchief
- handle any dressings or wounds
- make beds
- handle rubbish
- handle raw food
- handle dirty or soiled laundry.

When washing your hands it is important that you use the following technique, as this will remove most of the bacteria that cause contagious diseases (that is, diseases spread by direct or indirect contact).

Hand washing technique
- Wet your hands with hot running water
- Rub some liquid soap between your palms
- Rub your right palm over the back of your left hand
- Rub your left palm over the back of your right hand
- Rub your palms together with your fingers interlocked
- Rub the back of the fingers of your left hand with your right palm

- Rub the back of the fingers of your right hand with your left palm

- Rub around your left thumb with your right palm

- Rub around your right thumb with your left palm

- Rub your left fingertips round and round in your right palm

- Rub your right fingertips round and round in your left palm

- Rub your left wrist with your right hand

- Rub your right wrist with your left hand

- Rinse both hands thoroughly under running water

- Dry each hand on a clean paper towel

- Discard paper towel into pedal bin without touching the top or the sides of the bin

Remember: The correct hand washing procedure will take several minutes and you will still need to wash your hands even if you were wearing gloves.

Food that is not handled correctly can become contaminated with bacteria that cause food poisoning. Food poisoning bacteria grow in raw or waste food and rotting rubbish. Pests like mice and cockroaches carry food poisoning bacteria. Food poisoning bacteria are also carried by humans:

- *E. coli* is found in our intestines but is harmless to us until it comes into contact with food

- *Salmonella* may be found in raw meat, poultry, eggs, shellfish and faeces

- *Staphylococcus aureus* is found on our skin, in our nose, throat, mouth, ears, hair and nails, and in cuts and boils.

Most cases of food poisoning have an incubation period of between one and three days. This is the time it takes for symptoms to develop after eating contaminated food. The most common symptoms of food poisoning are:

- nausea

- vomiting

- diarrhoea.

Other symptoms of food poisoning include:

- stomach cramps

- abdominal pain

- loss of appetite

- a high temperature (fever) of 38°C (100.4°F) or above

- muscle pain and chills.

If care staff develop any of these symptoms they should not go to work. They should contact their manager for advice.

Most cases of food poisoning do not require medical attention, but you must contact the GP if service users have any of the following:

- vomiting that lasts for more than two days

- diarrhoea that lasts for more than three days

- blood in their vomit or stools

- any signs of dehydration.

Workplace procedures for safe food handling are governed by the Food Safety Act (1990) and the Food Safety (General Food Hygiene) Regulations (1995). For example, good personal hygiene is particularly important for preventing the spread of food poisoning bacteria. If you are involved in handling food, you should wash your hands with soap and hot running water before you handle food. You should also wash your hands after:

- handling any uncooked or waste food

- using the toilet

- assisting service users to use the toilet

- handling rubbish

- using or handling handkerchiefs or tissues

- coughing or sneezing

- touching your hair or face, or the hair and face of a service user.

If handling food, you should also:

- wear protective clothing

- keep your nails clean and short

- keep your hair tied back or covered

- cover any wounds with a coloured waterproof dressing

- not smoke in any area where food is being stored, prepared or served.

The spread of food poisoning bacteria can be controlled by cleaning and storing kitchen equipment correctly, in the following ways.

- Different surfaces should be used for preparing cooked and raw foods.

- Different equipment (knives, chopping boards etc) should be used for raw and cooked foods, and these should be kept separately.

- Work surfaces should be scrupulously cleaned after use for raw meat or poultry.

- All food should be kept covered.

- No food should be kept past its 'use-by' date.

The spread of food poisoning bacteria can also be controlled by cooking and storing food at the correct temperatures. Most bacteria are killed by heat at 70°C or above. Fridges and freezers should be set between -22 and five degrees centigrade, as most bacteria cannot reproduce at these temperatures. Be aware of food deteriorating too quickly – this may mean the fridge is not cold enough.

Always check 'use-by' dates on the food of service users who have a limited income as they may economise by buying produce with limited dates.

OTHER PERSONNEL WHO ASSIST INDIVIDUALS TO EAT AND DRINK

Kitchen staff

A large care home may require a chef to organise and oversee food production. Line cooks may be required to do the cooking and plating up. There also needs to be a dish washer to clean the dishes and peel vegetables. The dining area requires people to clear and set tables. In smaller care homes general kitchen staff will double up on these activities, for example, kitchen assistants may reheat food that has already been prepared for the evening meal.

All kitchen staff are required to have HACCP training. This stands for 'hazard analysis critical control point'. This is a system of food safety management that identifies the 'critical points' in a process where food safety problems (or 'hazards') could arise, and puts steps in place to prevent things from going wrong. Keeping records is an important part of HACCP, for example, checking and recording the core temperature of food before it is served.

The registered dietitian

A registered dietitian is able to assess, diagnose and treat diet and nutrition problems. They use the most up-to-date public health and scientific research on food, health and disease, which they translate into practical guidance to enable people to make appropriate lifestyle and food choices. Dietitians are regulated by the Health Professions Council and (like care workers) their work is governed by an ethical code to ensure that they always work to the highest standard. The title 'dietitian' can only be used by those appropriately trained professionals who are registered with the Health Professions Council. It is necessary to have a recognised degree, MSc or postgraduate diploma in nutrition and dietetics to work as a dietitian.

The speech and language therapist (SLT)

The medical term that is used to refer to difficulties with swallowing is dysphagia. Some people with dysphagia have problems swallowing certain foods or liquids, while others are completely unable to swallow. It is the speech and language therapist (SLT) who will make an initial assessment of these individuals and provide ongoing advice about treatment. SLTs are regulated by the Health Professions Council and (like care staff) are regulated by a code of practice, which is devised by the Royal College of Speech and Language Therapists. The SLT will identify whether an individual has the following.

- **Oropharyngeal or high dysphagia:** This is where the difficulties in swallowing are due to problems with the mouth or throat. These are often caused by problems with the nerves and muscles that help control the swallowing process.

- **Oesophageal or low dysphagia:** This is where the difficulties in swallowing are due to problems with the oesophagus (the tube that connects the mouth to the stomach). This is often caused by a blockage.

It is estimated that 30–40% of elderly people staying in nursing homes have some degree of dysphagia. It is a common complication of strokes, occurring in an estimated one in every two cases. Individuals who have dysphagia are at risk of malnutrition and dehydration. Also, difficulties with swallowing can mean that there is a chance that small particles of food or fluid can drop down (or be aspirated) into the lungs. This can cause a chest infection. The recommended treatment for dysphagia may include dietary modification or tube feeding (see **Chapter one**).

CASE STUDY: THE DIETITIAN

Mrs Smith is 72 years old and was admitted to the Laurels Nursing Home with dementia three months ago. Recently staff members have noticed that Mrs Smith has taken less interest in her food, and despite the best efforts of her relatives and care staff, she is starting to lose weight. In line with national and local guidance, staff carry out nutritional screening using the MUST tool each month. They have found that Mrs Smith's BMI is 18, and that her weight loss since admission is greater than 10%. Her overall MUST score is more than 2, meaning that Mrs Smith is at high risk of malnutrition. Staff members keep food charts for seven days, encourage nourishing snacks and drinks and fortify her food with high calorie and high protein ingredients. Mrs Smith is referred to the community dietitian for assessment and advice.

CASE STUDY: THE SPEECH AND LANGUAGE THERAPIST

Mrs Jones was admitted to Autumn Gardens Care Home three months ago for continuing health problems, having had several strokes in the past. She started to have trouble swallowing water without coughing and choking. A referral was made to the speech and language therapist who carried out a swallow assessment. The assessment found that part of Mrs Jones' brain responsible for controlling swallowing had been damaged during one of her strokes and that she is at risk of aspirating. The speech and language therapist recommended that all fluids are thickened before they are given to Mrs Jones, and that she must be supervised while she eats and drinks, as she is at significant risk of choking.

End of chapter quiz

1. What is BMI?

2. What is MUST? If an individual scored more than 2 on the MUST tool, what action would you take?

3. What is an SLT swallowing assessment?

4. What is oropharyngeal dysphagia?

5. What is HACCP?

6. Name three food poisoning bacteria.

7. Which professional body is responsible for regulating dietitians?

8. List three recommendations made by Age UK and the Royal College of Nursing for monitoring the dietary progress of service users.

9. List three principles of the Data Protection Act (1998) (DPA).

10. List three recommendations in *The Caldicott Report.*

My continuing professional development (CPD) log

Name of care worker ....

Name of manager/supervisor ....

Name of employer ....

Start date for training ....

Expected date of completion ....

This is to confirm that .... [*name of care worker*] has satisfactorily completed..................... [*insert number*] of hours of study, and has achieved all of the following learning points:

- Workplace policies and procedures that may influence the assessment of dietary need, for example, nutritional screening, person-centred approaches to care etc

- The monitoring of individual dietary therapies, for example, documentation and record keeping, observing and reporting, seeking guidance and advice etc

- The handling and serving of food to service users, for example, food hygiene, personal hygiene, assisted feeding etc

- Personnel who are involved in the nutrition and well-being of service users, for example, kitchen staff, speech therapists, dieticians etc

Comments from care worker or supervisor, for example, outcomes of key learning activities or results of quiz.

Signed (care worker): .... Date:............................

Signed (supervisor): .... Date:............................

Chapter three

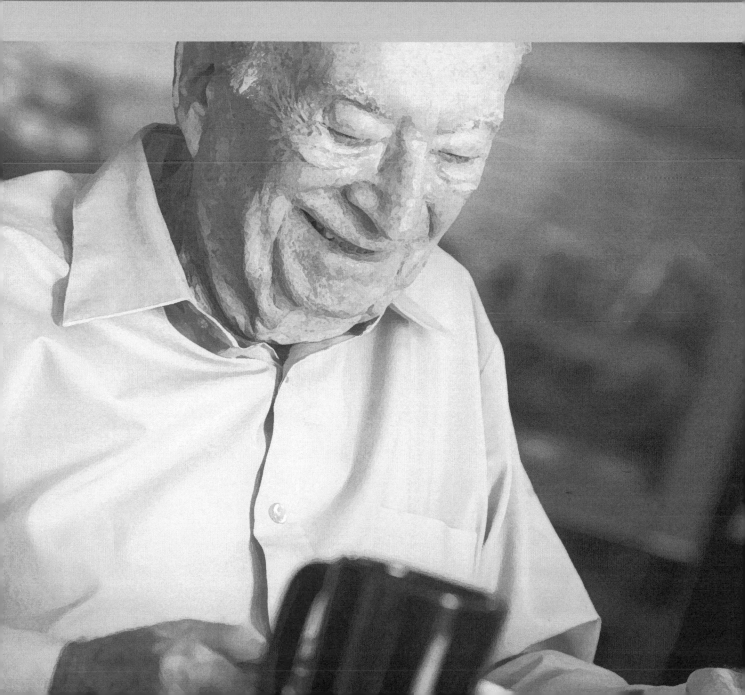

Chapter three

Diet and well-being

☺ Key learning activity

The following activities will provide you with key background information before you read **Chapter three**. Make a note of your answers and discuss these with a colleague or your supervisor before you start your reading.

Q1. How does the body use the following nutrients?

- Protein

- Carbohydrates

- Fats

- Minerals

- Vitamins

- Water

The following website will help you to complete this activity: www.nhs.uk/LiveWell/Goodfood/Pages/Goodfoodhome.aspx

Q2. The following activities draw on information provided by NHS Choices relating to the:

- factors influencing the purchase of food

- storage of food

- cooking and reheating of food.

The following website will help you to complete these activities: www.nhs.uk/LiveWell/Goodfood/Pages/Goodfoodhome.aspx

You can use the search facility in the top right-hand corner to look for key words such as 'food storage', 'food safety' etc.

a. What are the factors that influence you when buying food during your weekly shop?

b. What temperature should you set your refrigerator and freezer at?

c. Why does the food you buy have 'sell by' and 'use-by' dates written on the packaging?

d. What rules should you follow when reheating food?

AIMS OF THE CHAPTER

At the end of this chapter, the reader will have considered:

■ the constituents of a well balanced diet ie. water, carbohydrates, proteins, fats, minerals, vitamins and fibre

■ the factors that might influence purchasing food and drink, for example, nutritional values, cost and value for money etc

■ the importance of appropriate storage of food and drink, including carriage and delivery of foods and stock rotation, for example, cool box, refrigerator, freezer, larder etc

■ the importance of using the most appropriate method of cooking and reheating food for individuals within a residential or home care setting.

This chapter covers the underpinning knowledge for the following mandatory and optional units of the new Level 2 awards in food safety and nutrition (the number after refers to a learning outcome):

■ HSC 2029:3

■ HSC 2029:4

■ HSC 2029: 5

■ FSN 201:2

■ FSN 301:1

THE CONSTITUENTS OF A WELL BALANCED DIET

Food provides the body with energy so that it can carry out metabolic functions and be active. Food also provides essential nutrients for good health. A healthy diet allows us to:

■ grow, repair and replace cells and tissues within the body

■ produce energy for cell growth and the demands of physical activity

■ reduce risk of diseases such as heart disease and cancer.

A well balanced diet should contain the correct quantities of the following nutrients to meet our daily needs:

■ protein

■ carbohydrate

■ fats

■ minerals

■ vitamins

■ water.

Protein

Proteins are an essential nutrient for good health. They are used by the body for growth and the repair of cells and tissues. Proteins are made up of different amino acids. These amino acids combine to form the essential proteins that come from our food. All tissues in the body contain protein, including bone and hair. Enzymes and hormones are proteins and these are used in the body, for example, to digest food or control growth. Proteins also help messages to travel along nerve pathways and to assist muscles to contract. Some dietary sources of protein include meat, poultry, fish, eggs, milk, cheese, pulses, lentils, soya, nuts and tofu.

Carbohydrates

Carbohydrates provide an energy source for all systems of the body. Half of a person's total energy should come from carbohydrates. More active people, (for example, athletes), require a higher carbohydrate intake. Carbohydrates may be simple or complex. Simple carbohydrates include sugars such as glucose and fructose. Complex carbohydrates include starch and cellulose.

Carbohydrates are broken down by the body into glucose, which is then absorbed into the bloodstream to be transported to cells to provide them with the energy they require for metabolism. Sugars are digested and absorbed quickly, which can result in the so-called 'sugar rush', whereas complex carbohydrates are digested more slowly, resulting in a more constant release of glucose into the bloodstream. Complex carbohydrates can therefore help prevent hunger for longer periods.

As shown in the Eat Well Plate (see **Chapter one**) a third of our diet should be made up of sources of carbohydrates such as breakfast cereals, potatoes, rice, pasta, bread, pita bread and chapattis. Wholegrain varieties of these foods are a better choice since they are absorbed more slowly than white, refined versions and also contain more fibre.

Carbohydrates that are not used by the body are stored as glycogen and fat. When the diet provides insufficient energy in the form of calories, glycogen stores will be used as a source of energy. Once these stores have been used up, protein and fat will then be broken down to provide energy. To effectively break down fat, carbohydrates are required. If the diet is lacking in carbohydrate as well as total calories, the fat cannot be broken down properly and acidic chemicals called ketones are produced. This is called ketosis. Severe ketosis can alter the acidity of the blood, causing damage to the liver and kidneys.

Fats

Fats help us to make hormones, keep our skin healthy, and assist in maintaining the temperature of our body. They are therefore an important part of the diet. However, due to their high energy content, the amount of fat in the diet should be limited. It is recommended that fats should provide no more than 30% of our total daily energy intake.

Fats may be saturated or unsaturated. Saturated fats are usually solid at room temperature and mainly come from an animal source, for example, lard, cheese and butter. Too much saturated fat in our diet can increase our risk of developing heart disease or stroke, and can increase our risk of getting cancer. However, unsaturated fat can help to lower the levels of bad cholesterol (low density lipoproteins or LDL) in the blood and raise the level of good cholesterol (high density lipoproteins or HDL) in the blood, which can help to prevent heart disease and cancer. They also contain essential fatty acids that cannot be produced by the body, so are a necessary component of the diet in the correct quantities. Unsaturated fats are found in oily fish, such as salmon, trout and herring, sunflower and olive oils, avocados and some nuts and seeds.

Minerals

There are a number of minerals required by the body, each of which have varying functions from helping to build strong bones and teeth to helping to convert the food we eat into energy. The major minerals include the following.

Calcium is required for building strong bones and teeth, for blood clotting, and to help muscles and nerves to work. Low levels can result in osteoporosis. It is found in milk, cheese, some green vegetables, fish with edible bones, and foods made with calcium enriched flour, such as bread.

Iron has a number of roles in the body, such as helping to make the haemoglobin found in red blood cells. A deficiency of iron in the diet can result in iron-deficiency anaemia. Iron is found in meat, green leafy vegetables and fortified breakfast cereals.

Phosphorus is a component of bones and teeth. It is also involved in energy production within the cells of the body. Deficiency is rare but can cause symptoms such as weakness and joint pain. It is found in wholegrain cereals, fruit, meat, eggs and milk.

Magnesium has a number of important roles including maintaining muscle and nerve function, production and storage of energy and keeping bones strong. Severe deficiency can cause muscle cramps, palpitations and seizures. It is found in green leafy vegetables, nuts, bread, meat and dairy foods.

Sodium helps to regulate blood pressure and blood volume. It also helps with nerve transmission and muscle contraction. Many people have a diet that contains high levels of sodium, which can result in raised blood pressure. Deficiency can cause dizziness, confusion, muscle cramps and tiredness. Sodium is mainly found in salt, monosodium glutamate (MSG) and processed foods containing these ingredients. It is also present in eggs, meat, vegetables and milk.

Potassium helps the body to maintain fluid balance. It is also required for cell and nerve function and controls the acidity of the blood. Deficiency can cause an irregular heartbeat and muscle weakness. It is found in a number of foods including fruits, vegetables, milk, fish and nuts.

Vitamins

Vitamins are essential nutrients that are only needed in very small amounts and yet must be provided by our diet since our bodies cannot make enough of them for our needs. Vitamins may be fat soluble or water soluble. Fat soluble vitamins are mainly found in fatty foods such as vegetable oils, oily fish, butter and lard. They can easily be stored in the body and do not need to be eaten every day. Water soluble vitamins are found in fruit, grains and vegetables. However, water soluble vitamins can be easily destroyed by heat, and exposure to air, so we need to eat these regularly. Food containing water soluble vitamins should not be soaked in water. Nor should these foods be overcooked or kept hot for too long.

Some vitamins act as an antioxidant, meaning that they can help to protect cells by preventing damage caused by unstable molecules called free radicals, which are produced due to factors such as poor diet, smoking and radiation. Antioxidants are thought to lower the risk of developing cancer and heart disease. The main vitamins are as follows.

Vitamin A is a fat soluble vitamin and an antioxidant. It aids night vision and keeps skin healthy. Deficiency can cause night blindness, itching and dry skin. It is stored in the liver and can be harmful if eaten in excess. It is found in liver, fish oil, cheese, milk and eggs.

The **vitamin B** group are water soluble vitamins that include vitamin B1 (thiamin), vitamin B2 (riboflavin), vitamin B3 (niacin), vitamin B6 (pyridoxine), vitamin B12, pantothenic acid and folic acid. They are important for a healthy nervous system, production of haemoglobin and enabling energy to be released from the food we eat. Deficiency of vitamin B12 or folic acid can result in anaemia. They are found in meat, fish, eggs, fortified breakfast cereals, yeast extract, green vegetables, milk and wholegrains.

Vitamin C (ascorbic acid) is a water soluble vitamin and an antioxidant that is needed to keep cells and connective tissues healthy, so is important for wound healing. It also has a role in fighting infection and aiding the absorption of iron from plant sources in the diet. Vitamin C is not stored in the body, so sources need to be included in the diet every day. It is easily destroyed by heat and oxygen and is lost into the water if food is soaked. It can be preserved by using cooking methods such as steaming and stir frying. Although vitamin C is required in the diet daily, large doses should be avoided. Consuming amounts above the recommended daily dose does not improve the immune system or wound healing. In fact, excessive amounts can be harmful to health. Vitamin C deficiency may result in anaemia, poor healing, easy bruising and, in severe cases, scurvy. Vitamin C is found in a number of fruits and vegetables.

Vitamin D is a fat soluble vitamin that aids the absorption and regulation of calcium in the body. Deficiency can be difficult to identify in many cases since mild deficiency may have nil or non-specific symptoms. Vitamin D deficiency in childhood can result in rickets. Adults may complain of vague symptoms such as aches and pain. There are few food sources of vitamin D. It is found in oily fish, eggs, milk and vitamin D fortified foods. The main source of vitamin D for most people is that which is made in our own bodies when the skin is exposed to sunlight. Older people and people who are not exposed to sunlight should consider a vitamin D supplement.

Vitamin E is a fat soluble vitamin that plays an important antioxidant role in the body. It helps to keep cells healthy, therefore maintaining a healthy cardiovascular system and immune system. Deficiency is very rare, but can cause problems with the central nervous system. Vitamin E is found in sunflower oil, olive oil, nuts, spinach, tomatoes and wholegrain cereals.

Vitamin K is a fat soluble vitamin that is needed for blood clotting. Deficiency is very rare but can cause excessive bleeding. It is found in green leafy vegetables, olive oil and wholegrain cereals. It is also made by bacteria in the intestine.

Water

The human body is largely composed of water. We have water within our cells (intracellular) and outside of our cells (extracellular). It is essential for many of our bodily functions, such as carrying nutrients to and removing waste products from our cells, maintaining the structure of our cells and maintaining body temperature. Some of the water we consume is from the food we eat, but most of it is from the fluid we drink. Water is mainly absorbed by the jejunum (the middle section of the small intestine) and the colon. It is lost through perspiration and in our urine and faeces. The amount of water we need to consume depends upon factors such as our age, size and lifestyle, but most adults should aim to drink at least six to eight glasses of fluid each day.

Dehydration occurs when we drink insufficient fluid or if we lose too much fluid through vomiting, diarrhoea or sweating. Symptoms associated with mild dehydration include feeling thirsty, a dry mouth, concentrated urine, constipation, headaches and feeling tired. Chronic dehydration is when someone has been dehydrated over a long period of time. Symptoms include dry and chapped mouth, dry eyes, dry tongue, infrequent urination, constipation, fatigue, loss of appetite and, if severe, kidney problems and harm to the liver, joints and muscles. Severe dehydration is life-threatening, with symptoms such as low blood pressure, a weak pulse, seizures and loss of consciousness.

Older people are at risk of becoming dehydrated because they may not feel thirst as strongly as younger adults, they may choose to drink less so as to reduce the number of trips to the bathroom, they may have difficulty preparing and swallowing drinks, they may have poor kidney function or they may be taking medications that cause them to urinate more frequently. Older people should be encouraged and helped to drink regularly throughout the day, particularly if they are losing excess fluid, for example through vomiting, diarrhoea or perspiring because of a raised body temperature, or if they are showing signs of dehydration. Any symptoms of severe dehydration should be immediately reported to a healthcare professional.

FACTORS THAT INFLUENCE THE PURCHASE OF FOOD AND DRINK

As a care worker you might be involved in purchasing food on behalf of service users and you will, therefore, be expected to advise them on the cost and benefits of buying fresh, frozen or processed foods. As a consequence, you will need to know the different ways in which food is preserved and how this might affect the nutritional value of the food.

Fresh foods

The latest food guidelines recommend that adults eat at least five servings of fruit and vegetables every day. A serving of a fruit or vegetable is equal to:

■ one medium sized vegetable or fruit (such as an apple, orange or banana)

■ two small fruits (such as kiwi fruit or plums)

■ 80g of fresh, frozen or canned fruits or vegetables

■ 150ml fruit juice

■ a tablespoon of dried fruit

■ one bowl of green salad.

A diet rich in fresh fruit and vegetables lowers the risk of certain cancers, heart disease and other chronic diseases and conditions. Many fresh fruits and vegetables have high amounts of antioxidant vitamins, including vitamins A, C and E. In addition to their importance as a source of vitamins and minerals, fruits and vegetables also provide essential dietary fibre, which plays an important role in digestion, and is thought to have protective qualities against heart disease and some forms of cancer. Another benefit of fresh fruits and vegetables is their high water, low fat and low calorie nature. Fruits and vegetables contain very low levels of fats, and a diet low in fat can be effective for long-term weight loss.

Fresh fruits and vegetables have a lot of advantages besides just their nutritional importance. They come in a variety of colours, textures and flavours and can be used in virtually every meal. However, the vitamin content of fresh fruit and vegetables diminishes with age and can be destroyed by overcooking.

Processed foods

Processed foods (including canned and vacuum packaged meals) are generally treated or pre-prepared in some way, often for convenience, for example, ready meals. Although many people feel that processed foods are unhealthy, some processed foods are highly nutritious. For example, milk is a processed food because it is pasteurised to kill bacteria. Fruit and vegetable juices can also be an example of a healthy processed food. For example, some orange juices are fortified with vitamin C.

Of course, there are a lot of processed foods that aren't good for the person you are caring for. Many processed foods contain saturated fats and large amounts of salt and sugar. These types of foods should be avoided, or at least eaten sparingly. For example:

■ canned foods with lots of salt

■ packaged high calorie snack foods, like crisps and other fried snacks

■ high fat convenience foods, such as pizzas, pies and chips

■ packaged cakes and biscuits

■ sugary breakfast cereals

■ processed meats.

When the person is shopping for these foods, be sure to prompt them to look for products that are made with wholegrains, and which are low in salt and fat. Make sure you prompt them about serving size too, and to complement any processed foods they eat with some healthier choices such as fresh salad and wholegrain bread.

Frozen foods

Freezing is a way of preventing the growth of bacteria. The lack of moisture prevents bacteria from multiplying when the water freezes to ice and most bacteria become inactive at low temperatures. When fresh food is quick-frozen, the cold penetrates rapidly, freezing the water and forming small ice crystals. The smaller the ice crystals, the better the food quality will be after defrosting. If food is frozen slowly, larger ice crystals form. This means that as the water freezes and expands, the cell walls of the food expand and rupture, causing structural damage to the food. Therefore, the faster the food is frozen the better quality it will be, so make sure that you use the 'fast freeze' button on your freezer. If you don't have one, place the food at the bottom of the freezer, which is the coldest area, so that it freezes faster. Also, if you have several items to freeze, spread them out away from each other until they have completely frozen so they freeze quicker. The ideal temperature at which to store food items in the freezer for long periods of time is 0°F (-18°C) or lower.

Bacteria are not destroyed by the freezing process. Rather, they are just put out of action for the time that the food is frozen. However, as soon as the food begins to defrost, the temperature of the food rises and moisture is present, bacteria will start to grow. If the item is thawed at a temperature above 5°C bacteria will multiply rapidly in a very short time and this could lead to food poisoning.

Freezing does not lessen the nutritional value of the food. In fact, many frozen fruits and vegetables contain more nutrients than the fresh versions. This is because they are frozen straight after being picked, so nutrients are not lost through continued exposure to oxygen.

When freezing food you should:

■ ensure that food is in perfect condition before freezing

■ divide food into small portions as this aids rapid freezing

- use the correct type of packaging or container

- make sure that food is tightly wrapped or sealed, and that no air or water can get in or out

- check that the temperature of the freezer is at 0°F or below

- leave space around newly introduced packages

- defrost items in the refrigerator or in cold water.

Nutritional values

When nutritional information is given on a label, it must show the amount of each of the following in 100g or 100ml of the food:

- energy (in kJ and kcal)

- protein (in grams)

- carbohydrate (in grams)

- fat (in grams).

Some food products now have traffic light labels on the packaging, which show you at a glance if the food you are buying has high, medium or low levels of fat, saturated fat, sugars and salt. If you see a red light on the front of the pack you know the food is high in these nutrients. If you see amber, you know the food isn't high or low in these nutrients, but you might want to go for green. Green means that the food is low in that nutrient. The more green lights, the healthier the choice. Many of the foods with traffic light colours will have a mixture of red, amber and green. When you're choosing between similar products, try to go for more greens and ambers, and fewer reds, if you want to make the healthier choice. In addition to the traffic light system, you will also see the number of grams of fat, saturated fat, sugars and salt in a serving of the food.

You can find out more about the traffic light system at www.nhs.uk/livewell/goodfood/pages/food-labelling.aspx

Supporting individuals to work within a budget

As a care worker you may be working with people who are living on a limited budget. The following tips from www.moneybasics.co.uk/en/budget_and_banking/budgeting/reducing_spending.htm (moneybasics, 2011) will assist you to reduce the person's spending while you are shopping with them.

- Plan a menu together a week in advance and buy foods according to this.

- Consider bulk buying as this can save a lot of money.

- Always shop according to the person's list so that they are not tempted to buy unnecessary items.

- Visit supermarkets at the end of the day, when fresh food is often marked down in price.

- Look for own brand items in supermarkets as they are usually cheaper.

- When you get to the discount shelves (usually at the end of an aisle) see if there is anything you could purchase more cheaply.

- Buying fresh vegetables from the local market or greengrocer usually works out cheaper than buying from the supermarket.

- Buy fruit and vegetables that are in season.

- Watch the sell-by dates as you shop. You do not want to throw away food that you bought cheaply but cannot use in time.

- Use a calculator to keep a running total as you shop and check this against the till receipt – mistakes do occur.

- Take advantage of any money-off coupons you can.

Shopping safely

Food hygiene is not just important at home or in restaurants. You should also be aware of these principles when you are out shopping for food. You should:

- be aware of overloaded chilled or frozen food cabinets

- be aware of overly warm chilled or frozen food cabinets

- look to see if the shop assistant washes their hands carefully between handling raw and cooked foods s

- look to see if the shop assistant cleans or changes their utensils between handling raw and cooked foods

- not buy any packets that have been damaged or opened

- not buy food from counters where cooked and raw meat are not separated

- not delay getting chilled and frozen purchases home and into the correct storage as soon as possible to avoid defrosting or spoilage

- use a cool bag for carrying chilled or frozen purchases from the shops to the person's home.

STORAGE OF FOOD AND DRINK

If food is to remain in a good condition it must be stored correctly, in the right place and at the correct temperature for the appropriate period of time. As a care worker it is important for you to know how and where food should be stored to prevent food poisoning.

Storing food in the fridge

Some food needs to be kept in the fridge to help stop bacteria from growing. This includes:

- food with a use-by date

- cooked food

- ready to eat foods such as desserts and cooked meats.

Fridges should be kept between 0°C and 5°C, otherwise food poisoning bacteria will be able to grow. A fridge thermometer can be used to see whether it is at the right temperature. When using the fridge you should:

- keep the fridge door closed as much as possible

- wait for food to cool down before you put it in the fridge

- turn the temperature down if your fridge is full – to help keep it cold enough.

To help stop bacteria from growing you should:

- put any fresh food in the fridge and eat it within two days

- check the labels on jars and bottles to see if they need to be kept in the fridge once they have been opened

- keep food out of the fridge for the shortest possible time when you are preparing it – especially if the weather is warm

- keep prepared food, such as sandwiches, in the fridge until you are ready to eat them

- as a general rule, do not leave food out of the fridge for more than four hours

- cool leftovers as quickly as possible (ideally within one to two hours) and then store them in the fridge; eat any leftovers within two days, except for cooked rice, which you should eat within one day to help avoid food poisoning

- store raw meat and poultry in clean, sealed containers on the bottom shelf of the fridge, so that they don't touch or drip onto other food

- keep cooked meat separate from raw meat

- follow any storage instructions on the label and don't eat meat after its use-by date.

Storing food in the freezer

You can keep food safely in the freezer for years, as long as it has stayed frozen the whole time. However, the taste and texture of food changes if it is frozen for too long, so you might find that it's not very nice to eat. You can check any instructions on food labels or in your freezer's handbook to see how long food should be frozen. For safety, it is OK to freeze most raw or cooked foods providing you:

- freeze it before the use-by date

- follow any freezing or thawing instructions on the label

- thaw it in the fridge so that it doesn't get too warm

- use it within one to two days after it has been defrosted

- cook food until it is piping hot (steaming) all the way through.

When frozen meat thaws it produces lots of liquid. This liquid will contaminate any food, plates or surfaces that it touches. The thawed meat should be kept in a sealed container at the bottom of the fridge, so that it can't drip onto other foods. Plates, utensils, work surfaces and hands should be cleaned thoroughly after they have touched raw meat to stop bacteria from spreading. If you defrost raw meat and then cook it thoroughly, you can freeze it again, but you must never reheat food more than once.

Storing dry food

Dry foods include rice, pasta and flour, tinned foods, and unopened jars. You must keep loose food in sealed bags or containers. This helps to keep it fresh and stops anything falling into the food by accident. Also, you must:

- only reuse plastic water bottles if they are not damaged and you can clean them

- keep the storage area dry and cool

- not store food or drinks near cleaning products or other chemicals

- not use old food containers to store household chemicals

- not store food on the floor, because this will encourage rodents and other pests.

If you open a can of food and you are not going to use it all straightaway, empty the remaining food into a bowl, or other container, and put it in the fridge. You must not store food in an opened can, or re-use empty cans to cook or store food. This is because when a can has been opened and the food is open to the air, the tin from the can could contaminate the contents.

Cling film and kitchen foil

Cling film is useful for protecting food but you should check the instructions on the box to see what foods it can be used with. Bear in mind the following points when using cling film.

- Do not use cling film if it could melt into the food, such as in the oven or on pots and pans on the hob.

- You can use some types of cling film in the microwave, but make sure it doesn't touch the food.

- Only let cling film touch high fat foods when the instructions on the box says this is permissible.

Kitchen foil, made from aluminium, can be useful for wrapping and covering foods. However, you should not use foil or containers made from aluminium to store foods that are highly acidic, such as tomatoes, rhubarb and many types of soft fruit. This is because aluminium can be absorbed into the food if it is stored in contact with it for long periods of time.

'Best before' dates

'Best before' dates are found on frozen, dried, tinned and other foods. The best before date does not mean that the food will be harmful if eaten after the specified date, rather that it may lose its flavour and texture. However, you should not eat eggs after their best before date because eggs can contain *Salmonella* bacteria, which could multiply to high levels if you keep them after this date. The best before date will only be accurate if you have stored the food according to the instructions on the label.

Use-by dates

These appear on food that goes off quickly, for example, meat products and ready prepared salads. You shouldn't use any food or drink after the end of the use-by date on the label, even if it looks and smells fine. You must also follow the storage instructions. If you don't, the food will spoil more quickly and you will risk food poisoning. Use-by does not always mean eat-by. If the food can be frozen, its life can be extended beyond the use-by date. However, you must ensure that you follow any instructions on the pack, for example, 'freeze on the day of purchase'.

It is also important that you follow any instructions for cooking and preparation. Once a food with a use-by date has been opened, you will need to follow any instructions that are given, for example, 'eat within a week of opening'.

Display until dates

Date marks such as 'display until' or 'sell-by' appear next to the best before or use-by dates. They are used by staff to help with stock control and stock rotation.

METHODS OF COOKING AND REHEATING FOOD

Food that has been properly cooked should be steaming hot all the way through. To test this you should cut open the food and check that it is steaming hot in the middle. If you are cooking a large dish, you will need to check it in more than one place. Cooking thermometers or temperature probes are a more accurate way to check if food is cooked properly. The food should reach a temperature of 70°C for more than two minutes in the middle or thickest part.

Some foods change colour when they are cooked and checking the colour can sometimes be useful for determining whether foods such as meat are adequately cooked. It is very important to make sure that poultry, pork and meat products such as burgers, sausages and kebabs are properly cooked all the way through. If you are checking these foods you must cut into the middle and check that there is no pink meat left. The meat should also be steaming hot in the middle. If you are checking a whole chicken or other bird, pierce the thickest part of the leg with a clean knife or skewer until the juices run out. The juices shouldn't have any pink or red in them.

You can eat steaks and other whole cuts of beef and lamb rare, as long as the outside has been properly cooked or 'sealed'. Steaks are usually sealed in a frying pan over a high heat and this will kill any bacteria that might be on the outside. Pork joints and rolled joints shouldn't be served rare. To check these joints, you should put a skewer into the centre of the joint. The juices should not have any pink or red in them.

If you are not going to eat cooked food straightaway, you should cool it as quickly as possible and then store it in the fridge. Leftovers should not be kept for longer than two days. When you reheat food you must make sure that it is steaming hot all the way through. If the food is only warm it might not be safe to eat. Do not reheat food more than once.

End of chapter quiz

1. What is ketosis?

2. What are the symptoms of mild dehydration?

3. Why shouldn't you eat eggs after the 'best before' date?

4. What points should you remember when using cling film?

5. How do you know when food is properly cooked?

6. A serving of a fruit or vegetables is equal to...?

7. What should the temperature of a fridge be set at?

8. Milk is a processed food. True or false?

9. At what temperature should cooked food be served?

10. Bacteria are killed by freezing. True or false?

My continuing professional development (CPD) log

Name of care worker ....

Name of manager/supervisor ....

Name of employer ....

Start date for training...

Expected date of completion ....

This is to confirm that .... [*name of care worker*] has satisfactorily completed...................... [*insert number*] of hours of study, and has achieved all of the following learning points:

- The constituents of a well balanced diet ie. water, carbohydrates, proteins, fats, minerals, vitamins, fibre and water

- The factors that might influence purchasing food and drink, for example, nutritional values, food hygiene, cost and value for money etc

- The importance of appropriate storage of food and drink, including carriage and delivery of foods and stock rotation, for example, cool box, refrigerator, freezer, best by date, use-by date etc

- The importance of using the most appropriate method of cooking and reheating food for individuals within a residential or home care setting

Comments from care worker or supervisor, for example, outcomes of key learning activities or results of quiz.

Signed (care worker): .... Date:............................

Signed (supervisor): .... Date:............................

Chapter four

Legislation and guidance related to food and drink

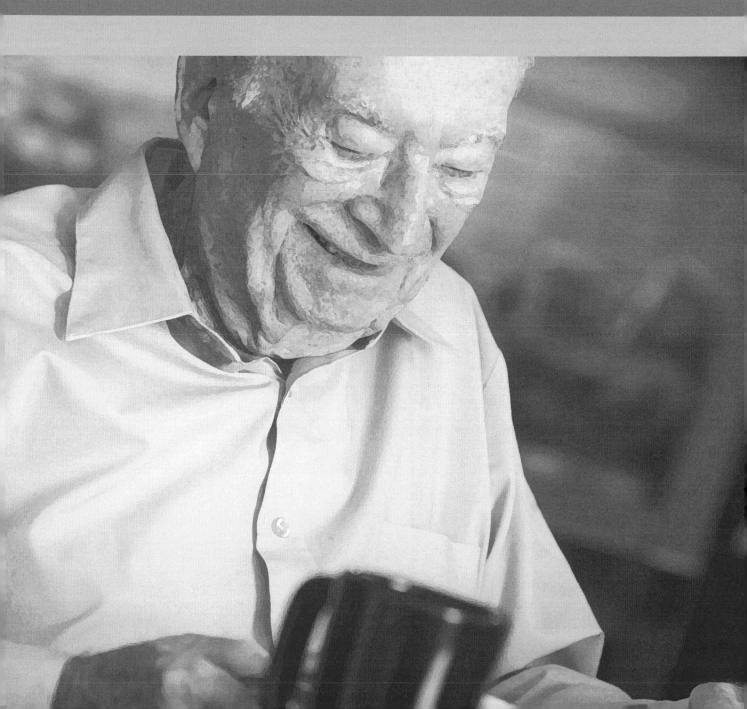

Chapter four

Legislation and guidance related to food and drink

☺ Key learning activity

The following instructions outline the responsibility of employers and employees under the Health and Safety at Work Act (1974). For each of the following responsibilities give one example that is relevant to food and drink.

Q1. Carry out risk assessments

Q2. Ensure health and safety regulations are observed

Q3. Provide safety equipment

Q4. Ensure staff are properly trained

Q5. Report injuries, diseases and dangerous occurrences to the appropriate authority

Q6. Use the equipment that is provided properly

Q7. Report hazards

Q8. Take care of your own and other people's safety

Q9. Attend health and safety training

Q10. Follow policies and procedures

Make a note of your answers and discuss these with a colleague or your supervisor before you start your reading.

AIMS OF THE CHAPTER

At the end of this chapter, the reader will have considered the:

■ specific legislation, regulations and guidance that govern nutrition and food preparation and handling, for example, the Health and Safety at Work Act (1974), the Food Safety Act (1990), the Food Safety (General Food Hygiene) Regulations etc

■ organisation's workplace policies and procedures governing nutrition and well-being, food and drink preparation, and presentation.

This chapter covers the underpinning knowledge for the following Level 2 mandatory units in food safety and nutrition.

- HSC 2029: 1
- HSC 209: 2
- HSC 209: 3
- HSC 209: 4
- HSC 209: 5
- HSC 209: 6

LEGISLATION AND REGULATIONS

The Health and Safety at Work Act (1974)

Through this act of parliament, the Health and Safety Commission (HSC) and the Health and Safety Executive (HSE) were formed to monitor safety in the workplace. The HSC is responsible for proposing new regulations to the government and the HSE is responsible for the enforcement of this law. The HSE does this by sending out inspectors to monitor whether health and safety regulations are being implemented in the workplace and if they are not, the inspectors have a wide range of powers that they can use. The act aims to meet the following requirements:

1. to protect all people who work in your premises and any other people who visit your workplace

2. to protect the health, safety and welfare of all employees, whether they are full-time or part-time

3. to protect all employees who may be exposed to risk in their workplace activity.

The act is the basis for all current food safety and food hygiene legislation and aims to safeguard the health, safety and welfare of all workers and all those in employment.

According to the act, an employer must:

- make the workplace safe and free from risk to health
- assess risks and take action to reduce them
- devise a health and safety policy and ensure that all employees are aware of it
- provide training, information and supervision to employees
- provide adequate first aid and welfare facilities
- provide protective equipment and clothing free of charge
- have emergency procedures in place

- assess dangers, and take precautions and provide safety signs

- avoid the risk from injury from manual handling operations

- report injuries, diseases and dangerous occurrences to the appropriate authority.

The employer must take action that 'is reasonably practicable' and preventative measures need to be taken before an accident occurs, rather than implemented after an accident occurs.

All changes to workplace health and safety regulations must be disseminated to employees by the health and safety representative or safety committee, to ensure that the employees are kept up-to-date with current practice. The company's health and safety policy should also reflect any current changes to legislation.

The Health and Safety at Work Act (1974) influences many working practices, including:

- provision of protective equipment and safe working practice

- procedures for storing, movement and use of substances and materials

- welfare facilities ie. toilets, washing facilities, restrooms etc

- training in health and safety legislation

- identification of areas of risk and control of risk procedures

- first aid facilities

- emergency procedures

- clear rules that outline individual responsibilities

- proper maintenance of equipment

- control of exposure to harmful substances

- manual handling operations

- monitoring of injuries, diseases and dangerous occurrences

- provision of safety signs

- provision of protective clothing and equipment free of charge

- reduced danger from fire, noise, electrical equipment etc

- satisfactory provision of ventilation, temperature, lighting, sanitary and washing facilities, rest facilities

- clearly signed emergency exits.

Under the Health and Safety at Work Act (1974), employees must ensure that they:

- take care of their own health and safety and that of others who they work with

- co-operate with their employer's policies and procedures

- use equipment correctly in accordance with the appropriate instructions and training

- do not tamper with or misuse anything that is provided by their employer for their health, safety and welfare

- participate in health and safety training

- report any hazards or risks

- keep current and up-to-date with health and safety issues

- wear protective equipment and protective clothing when required.

It is essential for all employees to be trained in the use of workplace equipment and how to use it safely, and to ensure that any faults in the equipment are reported to the manager or health and safety representative. Employees must follow their company's policies and procedures in relation to health and safety in the workplace

The Food Safety Act (1990)

The Food Safety Act (1990) affects everyone who works in the production, processing, storage, distribution and sale of food. The act aims to ensure that all food produced for sale is safe to eat, meets quality expectations and is not presented in a misleading way. It also provides legal powers and penalties.

The act is enforced by environmental health officers working for local governments who have powers to enable them to enforce the act. The food safety requirements are that food throughout the food chain must not:

- have been rendered injurious to health

- be unfit or so contaminated that it would be unreasonable to expect it to be eaten.

Food Safety (General Food Hygiene) Regulations (1995)

These regulations provide the legal requirements that care organisations are required to fulfill. When inspecting premises, environmental health officers are looking for compliance with these regulations. The basic requirements of the regulations are outlined by Solihull Metropolitan Council (2010a), as follows:

	Food Safety (General Food Hygiene) Regulations (1995)	Recommendation/advice
Structure/ cleanliness	Food premises must be kept clean and maintained in a good condition and state of repair to permit adequate cleaning and disinfection. The walls, floors, ceilings, doors, windows and food contact surfaces in all food premises must be maintained, in good repair and condition to permit adequate cleaning/ disinfection with no danger of contamination by external sources such as pests. Drainage facilities must be adequate and they must be designed and constructed to avoid the risk of contamination of food stuffs.	'Clean as you go'– it is recommended you implement an effective cleaning schedule to cover all of the premises and all equipment within it. The type of material used that is suitable for surfaces will depend upon the activity in each room. It is recommended that areas which are subject to intense use are finished to provide a more durable surface. Use a cleaning schedule. Direction of flow from clean to dirty areas. Grids should be easy to clean.
Lighting/ ventilation	Adequate ventilation (mechanical or natural) must be provided to ensure that heat and/or humidity do not build up to levels that could compromise food safety. The air must not flow from a contaminated area to a clean area. All parts of the ventilation system, including filters, must be accessible for cleaning and maintenance. Adequate natural and/or artificial lighting must be provided to all areas of the food premises to allow safe food handling, effective cleaning and monitoring of cleaning standards.	As a target, ambient temperatures should be below 25°C. Natural ventilation will only be suitable for small premises. The levels of lighting should be enough to ensure that the work can be carried out easily and safely. Glass lights should be protected with shatterproof diffusers in areas where open food is handled.
Sanitary conveniences	An adequate number of suitable toilets must be readily available and they must not lead directly into any room where food is handled. Toilets must have either natural or mechanical ventilation.	Mechanical systems should discharge away from food rooms.

	Food Safety (General Food Hygiene) Regulations (1995)	**Recommendation/advice**
Hand wash basin	An adequate number of designated hand wash basins must be readily available. The hand washing basins must be provided with: ■ hot and cold (or appropriately mixed) running water ■ materials for cleaning the hands ■ materials for drying the hands. Where necessary, the provision for washing food must be kept separate from the hand washing facility.	The need for regular hand washing must be considered, particularly where both raw and cooked foods are handled. Warm water should be approximately 45°C. It is good practice to use antibacterial soap from a dispenser. It is not recommended that a towel that can be used on the same part twice is used. It is good practice to display signs to identify designated 'hand wash' basins. Nail brushes must be kept clean.
Changing facilities	Adequate changing facilities for staff must be provided where necessary eg. depending upon the size and type of the business and the number of employees, to allow separate storage of street clothes and personal items.	Personal lockers for staff are recommended.
Washing equipment	Where necessary, adequate facilities must be provided for washing equipment. The facilities must be constructed of materials resistant to corrosion and must be easy to clean and have an adequate supply of hot and cold water.	Twin sinks are preferable, to allow washing and rinsing.
Washing food	Where necessary, adequate facilities must be made for washing food, although one sink may be used for washing both food and equipment in smaller operations. Sinks for washing food must be provided with a supply of hot and/or cold running water, and must be kept clean.	It is good practice to display signs to indicate the use of the sink. Where the same sink is used for washing food and equipment, time separation should be used to separate the operations and the sink should be disinfected between uses.

Nutrition and Well-being for Vulnerable Adults © Pavilion Publishing (Brighton) Ltd 2012

	Food Safety (General Food Hygiene) Regulations (1995)	Recommendation/advice
Equipment	All items that come into contact with food, including packaging, must be kept clean, be in good condition and made of suitable material so as to minimise the risk of contamination. You must ensure that equipment will be thoroughly cleaned and, where necessary, disinfected and be installed so that the surrounding area can be adequately cleaned.	The equipment you choose should be suitable for the job. It should be non-toxic, smooth, inert to both food and cleaning materials and capable of being cleaned and disinfected. Implement a cleaning schedule. Separate surfaces/equipment should be used to reduce the risk of cross-contamination from raw to cooked foods.
Personal hygiene	Every person working in a food handling area must maintain a high degree of personal cleanliness and where appropriate wear suitable, clean clothing. No person known or suspected to be a carrier of a disease that can be passed on by food (eg. infected wounds, skin infections, diarrhoea, vomiting) may work in any food handling area if there is a possibility of contaminating the food. If you are suffering from any of the above or a member of your family is suffering from diarrhoea/vomiting you must inform your manager immediately.	Changing facilities for staff. No smoking. Provide adequate clothing eg. uniform, hat, hairnet. Implement personal hygiene policies. Implement a return to work policy to include: ■ return to work after holiday ■ pre-employment questionnaire ■ return to work after illness. This should inform staff of their duties. Ensure that clearance from the doctor is gained before allowing a member of staff to return to work after illness.

	Food Safety (General Food Hygiene) Regulations (1995)	Recommendation/advice
Food waste	Food waste must not be allowed to accumulate in food rooms. Food waste and other refuse must be deposited in closable containers, which are easy to clean and disinfect. Adequate provision must be made for the removal and storage of food waste and other refuse. Refuse stores must be designed and managed to enable them to be kept clean, to prevent access by pests and against contamination of food, drinking water, equipment or premises.	It is good practice to remove all waste from the food room at the end of the day. Cleaning schedules should ensure that the lined, refuse containers are regularly cleaned and disinfected inside and out. Outdoor storage areas should not be next to the delivery entrance. It is recommended that the refuse area is well lit and that it has a hose for cleaning and draining.
Water supply	There must be an adequate supply of potable water to ensure that food does not become contaminated. Potable water must be used: ■ for the cleaning of food ■ for inclusion in food recipes ■ for cleaning of food equipment	Generally, it can be assumed that water will be potable if it comes from a main water supply. Ice for drinks should not be handled with bare hands and glassware should not be used for shovelling ice.
	■ for cleaning of surfaces in contact with food ■ for hand washing. Ice must be made from potable water, where possible, to ensure it does not contaminate food.	
Hazard analysis	Operators of a food business must assess the processes in their business, identify any possible hazards, and decide how these can be reduced or eliminated so that the end product is safe. Having assessed the hazards and introduced controls, the hazards should be monitored regularly and amended as necessary. This is known as hazard analysis.	Although it is not a legal requirement to document your hazard analysis, it is recommended that you do. This will help you to demonstrate that you have identified hazards which exist in your business and methods for their control.

Information adapted with permission from the Solihull Metropolitan Council website (2010a)

The Food Hygiene Regulations (2006)

These regulations apply to temperature control. In the care home these might apply to the:

■ preparation of food

■ handling of food

■ storage of food

■ transporting of food, for example, to the table.

There are a number of food types that are subject to temperature control. Including:

■ cooked products and ready to eat products

■ dairy products

■ smoked or cured ready to eat meat and fish and some raw fish

■ fresh pasta and uncooked/partly cooked pasta and dough products.

The Solihull Metropolitan Council website (2010b) includes a table that shows the basic requirements of the legislation.

	The Food Hygiene Regulations (2006)	Recommendation/advice
Chilled food	Food may not be stored at a temperature above 8°C if it is likely to support the growth of pathogenic organisms or the formation of toxins.	Regularly check the temperature of all refrigerators to ensure that they are operating below 8°C and record this check.
	If a lower storage temperature is specified by the manufacturer, the food must be stored at that lower temperature, provided it is necessary for the safety of the food.	Check the manufacturer's storage guidelines upon receipt of the food and ensure that the guidelines are followed.
	Cold food on display for service can be out of temperature control for one period up to a maximum of four hours. After the four-hour period has expired, food must be stored under temperature control or discarded.	Any item of food can be displayed out of temperature control only once. It is good practice to record when the food went on display and when it had finished being displayed, as the burden of proof is upon the caterer.

	The Food Hygiene Regulations (2006)	Recommendation
Hot cooked/ reheated food		It is good practice to check the temperature of hot, reheated or cooked food using a calibrated temperature probe to ensure it has reached a temperature that will destroy pathogenic micro-organisms. The FSA recommends that food is cooked to a temperature of 70°C for two minutes, or an equivalent temperature and time eg. 75°C for 30 seconds.

It is recommended that you record cooking or reheated food temperatures. |
| **Hot-hold food** | Hot food should be displayed or stored at a temperature of 63°C or above.

Food may be kept at a temperature cooler than 63°C for one period of up to a maximum of two hours if it is for service or display. | It is good practice to monitor and record the temperature of food during the display period, using a calibrated thermometer to ensure that it is above 63°C.

If the food is kept below 63°C it is advisable to record when the food was put on display and when it was taken off display as the burden of proof is on the caterer. |

Information adapted with permission from the Solihull Metropolitan Council website (2010b)

The Care Quality Commission

The Care Quality Commission (CQC) is an independent agency set up by the government as a result of the Health and Social Care Act (2008). It promotes improvements and ensures quality standards are being met. It reports to the government and publishes a report to parliament on the state of social care.

The CQC regulates, inspects and reviews all adult social care services in the public, private and voluntary sectors in England. This includes:

- care homes for older people (65+)

- care homes for adults (18 to 65)

- domiciliary care (home care).

The inspection system that is used puts people who use care services and their views at the heart of how they judge the quality of services. This allows the CQC to:

- include people who use services in the inspection teams

- arrive unannounced and carry out an inspection

- focus on improving services

- be tough on care providers who fail to meet minimum standards

- make reports easy for everyone to read.

The CQC has a quality rating in place for all care providers ranging from zero stars (poor) to three stars (excellent)

The regulation of care homes is measured against the standards contained within Regulation 14 of the Health and Social Care Act (2008) (Regulated Activities) Regulations 2010 and with regard to nutrition these state the following.

1. *'Where food and hydration are provided to service users as a component of the carrying on of the regulated activity, the registered person must ensure that service users are protected from the risks of inadequate nutrition and dehydration, by means of the provision of –*

    a. *a choice of suitable and nutritious food and hydration, in sufficient quantities to meet service users' needs;*

    b. *food and hydration that meet any reasonable requirements arising from a service user's religious or cultural background; and*

    c. *support, where necessary, for the purposes of enabling service users to eat and drink sufficient amounts for their needs.*

2. *For the purposes of this regulation, "food and hydration" includes, where applicable, parenteral nutrition and the administration of dietary supplements where prescribed.'*

POLICY AND PROCEDURE

Care homes are required to develop policies, procedures and codes of practice on food safety, nutrition and food hygiene. They must keep detailed records so that their inspector can identify whether the meals served meet the above standards and check that special diets are catered for. Records must also show that the best principles of food hygiene are practiced. For example, environmental health inspectors will want to examine the records for monitoring the temperature of food that is stored – so records of fridge and freezer temperatures must be maintained on a daily basis. Your employer is required to develop organisational policies and procedures that comply with the food safety legislation discussed in this chapter. This will include:

- food storage

- food preparation

- cleaning procedures

- waste disposal

- personal hygiene of staff

- record keeping

- staff training.

In addition to this, your employer is required by the CQC to develop food and nutrition policies that cover topics such as:

- nutritional needs assessment

- how and where to refer those who are at risk of malnutrition

- the minimum standards expected for the provision of food and drink

- how staff are introduced to and trained in good practice

- how eating and drinking records are maintained.

An example of a nutrition policy is given in **Appendix B**.

In the study *Still Hungry to Be Heard*, Age UK (2010) highlights the problems of malnutrition in older people as follows.

- Malnutrition affects people in later life more than anyone else.

- Malnutrition affects 32% of people over the age of 65.

- People who are admitted to hospital over the age of 80 are twice as likely to become malnourished than those under the age of 50.

- Becoming malnourished leads to serious consequences, such as staying in hospital for longer, taking more medications, an increased risk of suffering from infections and even death.

- Malnutrition costs the NHS and the taxpayer a lot of money.

In order for malnutrition in hospitals to be addressed, Age UK recommends that organisations responsible for delivering healthcare implement the following steps.

- Hospital staff must listen to patients, their relatives and carers, and respond to what they say. Ward staff should ask patients about their needs at mealtimes, such as food preferences, any difficulties with eating and their appetite, and ensure these are met.

- All ward staff must become food aware. Ward staff need to understand that every meal is important; it is not acceptable for patients to miss meals. Ward staff must follow their own professional codes and guidance from other bodies.

■ Organisations responsible for healthcare delivery need to ensure they are fulfilling the Department of Health's core standards on food and help with eating. People should be offered food that is suitable to their needs as well as given assistance to eat. It is important to maintain dignity around meals, such as offering napkins rather than bibs and assisting people to eat with cutlery where possible.

The Royal College of Nursing's Nutrition Now campaign aims to raise standards of nutrition and hydration in hospitals and the community. Nutrition and hydration are considered to be as essential to care as medication and other types of treatment.

Care staff must assess patients for the signs or risk of malnutrition on admission and at regular intervals during their hospital stay. All patients should be screened upon arrival for any signs of malnutrition. Regular screening allows care staff to determine whether a person's nutritional status is improving or not. Staff members need to understand the importance of screening and how to complete the screening tool correctly.

Hospitals and care homes should introduce 'protected mealtimes'. When mealtimes are protected, it means that all non-urgent activity must stop. This allows the people being cared for to eat their meals and makes sure that care workers have the time to assist them.

Hospitals and care homes should implement a 'red tray' system and ensure that it works in practice. The use of a coloured tray can help care staff members to identify which patients need assistance with their meal.

Hospitals and care homes should use trained volunteers where appropriate. Volunteers can provide further assistance at mealtimes, such as helping to cut up food, making sure food is within reach or providing company during the meal.

Although originally intended for hospitals, these recommendations are useful in other organisations where food is provided. To what extent do you feel that your organisation follows these recommendations?

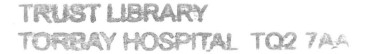

☺ Key learning activity: Developing a code of practice for assisting an individual to eat and drink

To what extent do you feel that your organisation has implemented the following recommendations? Please give specific examples.

- Service users are consulted about menus, their meal requirements and their food preferences.

- All care staff are food aware.

- Service users are screened to determine whether they are at risk of malnutrition upon admission and at regular intervals during their stay.

- Protected mealtimes have been introduced.

- Those at nutritional risk are identified on admission and a system put in place to signal the need for help, for example, 'red tray'.

- Volunteers are used, where appropriate, to assist service users at mealtimes.

End of chapter quiz

1. What are the general requirements of the Health and Safety at Work Act (1974)?

2. Which local authority officer is responsible for ensuring compliance with the Food Safety Act (1990)?

3. Which food types are subject to temperature control?

4. What is the Care Quality Commission?

5. What do the CQC Essential Standards of Quality and Safety say about the use of menus?

6. List three factors that a food safety policy should cover.

7. List three things that a nutrition policy should cover.

8. What are protected mealtimes?

9. What is the 'red tray' system?

10. What is of paramount importance in implementing a 'red tray' system?

✑ My continuing professional development (CPD) log

Name of care worker ....

Name of manager/supervisor ....

Name of employer ....

Start date for training..

Expected date of completion ....

This is to confirm that .... [*name of care worker*] has satisfactorily completed...................... [*insert number*] of hours of study, and has achieved all of the following learning points:

■ Legislation, regulations and guidance that govern nutrition and food preparation and handling, for example, the Food Safety Act (1990), the Care Standards Act (2000) etc

■ The organisation's workplace policies and procedures governing nutrition and well-being, food and drink preparation, and presentation

Comments from care worker or supervisor, for example, outcomes of key learning activities or results of quiz.

Signed (care worker): .... Date:................................

Signed (supervisor): .... Date:................................

References

Age Concern and The Royal College of Nursing (2007a) *Helping an Older Person to Eat* [online]. London: Age Concern. Available at: www.ageuk.org.uk/Documents/EN-GB/helping%20an%20older%20person%20to%20eat%20leaflet.pdf?dtrk=true (accessed November 2011).

Age Concern and The Royal College of Nursing (2007b) *Is an Older Person you Care About Malnourished?* [online]. London: Age Concern. Available at: www.dignityincare.org.uk/_library/Resources/Dignity/CSIPComment/signs_of_malnutrition_leaflet.pdf (accessed November 2011).

Age UK (2010) *Still Hungry to Be Heard: The scandal of people in later life becoming malnourished in hospital.* London: Age UK.

British Association for Parenteral and Enteral Nutrition (undated) *The MUST Report. Nutritional screening of adults: A multidisciplinary responsibility* [online]. Available at: www.bapen.org.uk/must_report.html (accessed March 2010).

CancerHelp UK (2010a) *Percutaneous Endoscopic Gastrostomy Feed* [online]. Available at: www.cancerhelp.org.uk/coping-with-cancer/coping-physically/diet/managing/drip-or-tube-feeding (accessed February 2010).

Cancer Help UK (2010b) *Detailed Diagram of a Percutaneous Endoscopic Gastrostomy (PEG) Feeding Tube* [online]. Available at: www.cancerhelp.org.uk/coping-with-cancer/coping-physically/diet/managing/drip-or-tube-feeding (accessed February 2010).

Care Quality Commission (2010) *Guidance about Compliance: Essential standards of quality and safety.* London: Care Quality Commission.

Department of Health (1995) *The Caldicott Committee: Report on the review of patient-identifiable information.* London: Department of Health.

Department of Health (2003) *Confidentiality: NHS Code of Practice.* London: Department of Health.

Gregory J (2000) *The National Diet and Nutrition Survey: Young people aged 4 to 18 years. Vol 1: Report of the diet and nutrition survey.* London: Office for National Statistics.

Harbottle L (2007) *Healthy Eating and Depression: How diet may help protect your mental health.* London: Mental Health Foundation.

Henderson L, Gregory J, Irving K & Swan G (2003) *The National Diet and Nutrition Survey: Adults aged 19 to 64 years. Vol 2: Energy, protein, carbohydrate, fat and alcohol intake.* London: Office for National Statistics.

Mental Health Foundation (2007) *Healthy Eating and Depression* [online]. Available at: www.mentalhealth.org.uk/content/assets/PDF/publications/healthy_eating_depression.pdf (accessed October 2011).

Moneybasics (2011) *Tips to Reduce Spending* [online]. Available at: www.money basics.co.uk/en/buget_and_banking/budgeting/reducing_spending.html (accessed December 2011).

National Institute for Health and Clinical Excellence (2006) *Nutrition Support for Adults: Oral nutrition support, enteral tube feeding and parenteral nutrition.* London: NICE.

NHS Choices (a) *The Eatwell Plate* [online]. Available at: www.nhs.uk/livewell/goodfood/pages/eatwell-plate.aspx (accessed October 2011).

NHS Choices (b) *Live Well* [online]. Available at: www.nhs.uk/livewell/healthy-eating/Pages/Healthyeating.aspx (accessed October 2011).

NHS Choices (c) Birth to Five: Vitamins [online]. Available at: www.nhs.uk/Planners/birthtofive/Pages/Vitamins.aspx (accessed October 2011).

NHS Choices (d) *Why Breastfeed?* [online]. Available at: www.nhs.uk/planners/breastfeeding/pages/why-breastfeed.aspx (accessed October 2011).

NHS Choices (e) Introducing Solid Foods: The first steps [online]. Available at: www.nhs.uk/planners/birthtofive/pages/weaningfirststeps.aspx (accessed October 2011).

Office of Public Sector Information (1998) *The Data Protection Act.* London: OPSI. .

Solihull Metropolitan Council (2010a) *Food Business: Food safety regulations (general hygiene requirements for all)* [online]. Available at: www.solihull.gov.uk/business/generalhygiene.htm (accessed March 2010).

Solihull Metropolitan Council (2010b) *Food Business: Food safety regulations (temperature control required for food)* [online]. Available at: www.solihull.gov.uk/business/temperaturecontrol.htm (accessed March 2010).

Appendix A

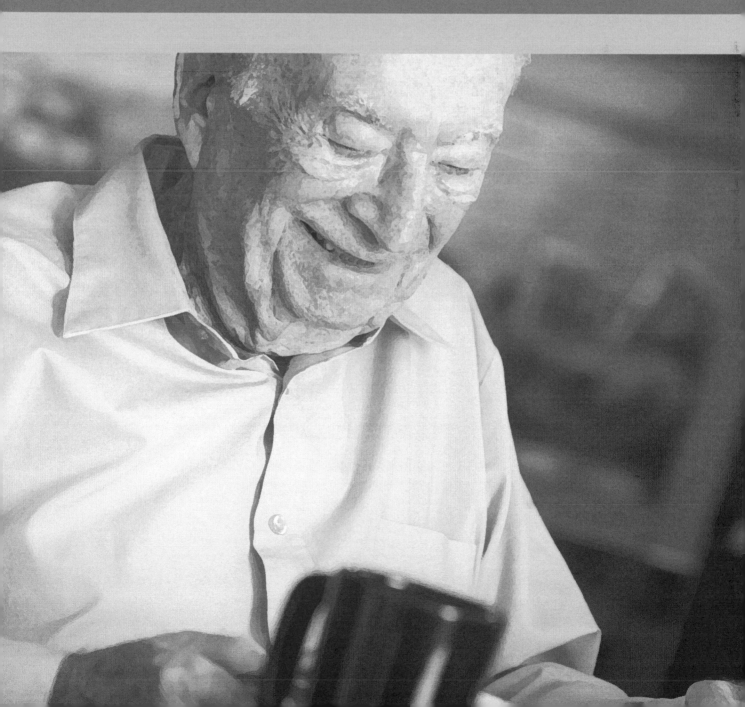

End of chapter quiz answers

CHAPTER ONE ANSWERS

Q1. List six essential nutrients for a healthy diet.
Protein, carbohydrate, fats, minerals, vitamins, fibre and water

Q2. Outline the eight healthy eating tips recommended by the NHS Choices *Live Well* website
1. Meals should be based on starchy foods
2. Eat more fruit and vegetables
3. Eat more fish
4. Cut down on saturated fat and sugar
5. Eat less salt
6. Drink plenty of water
7. Do not miss breakfast
8. Be active and try to be a healthy weight

Q3. Why is iron needed in the body?
This mineral helps to keep red blood cells healthy. Insufficient intake can lead to anaemia.

Q4. Give three risk factors for premature death in adults.
- Raised blood cholesterol
- Raised blood pressure
- Obesity
- Physical inactivity
- Excessive alcohol intake

Q5. How might these risk factors be limited through diet?
Reduce the intake of saturated fats, sugar, salt and alcohol, and eat at least five portions of fruit and vegetables a day.

Q6. How might you alter the diet for an older person to compensate for weight loss?
Offer nourishing snacks, offer nourishing drinks, and fortify foods with high calorie and high protein ingredients.

Q7. What is osteoporosis?
Thinning of the bones due to excessive calcium loss

Q8. How might you increase dietary intake of calcium?
Ensure that calcium rich foods (such as milk, yoghurt, cheese, calcium enriched soya milk and fish containing edible bones) are eaten every day. Calcium supplements may be necessary for people who dislike or cannot tolerate these foods.

Q9. What are the risks associated with PEG feeding?

The risks include reflux and regurgitation of the feed with possible aspiration into the lungs. This could cause a chest infection.

Q10. What position should a person receiving a PEG feed be nursed in?

Sitting up at an angle of at least 45 degrees

CHAPTER TWO ANSWERS

Q1. What is BMI?

Body mass index is a measure using height and weight to identify whether an adult is a healthy weight, or is over or underweight.

Q2. What is MUST? If an individual scored more than 2 on the MUST tool, what action would you take?

MUST is the Malnutrition Universal Screening Tool. If an individual scores more than 2 on the MUST tool, you should follow local nutrition policy or guidelines and consider referral to a dietitian.

Q3. What is an SLT swallowing assessment?

A speech and language therapy swallowing assessment will determine a service user's degree of swallowing difficulty

Q4. What is oropharyngea dysphagia?

This is where the difficulties in swallowing are due to problems with the mouth or throat. These are often caused by problems with the nerves and muscles that help control the swallowing process. It is common among individuals who have had a stroke.

Q5. What is HACCP?

HACCP stands for hazard analysis critical control point. This is a system of food safety management that identifies the 'critical points' in a process where food safety problems (or 'hazards') could arise, and puts steps in place to prevent things from going wrong.

Q6. Name three food poisoning bacteria.

E.coli, *Salmonella* and *Staphylococcus aureus*

Q7. Which professional body is responsible for regulating dietitians?

The Health Professions Council

Q8. List three recommendations made by Age UK and the Royal College of Nursing for monitoring the dietary progress of service users.

Care workers should check for, record, and report:

- any significant weight loss
- any recent loss of appetite
- any loose fitting clothes
- signs of recurrent infections and any difficulty recovering from illness

- any loss of ability to keep warm
- constipation or diarrhoea
- pressure sores
- any ill-fitting dentures, or swollen or bleeding gums
- sore mouth or tongue
- difficulties chewing or swallowing
- tooth decay.

Q9. List three principles of the Data Protection Act (1998) (DPA).

Personal data should:
- be obtained fairly and lawfully
- be held for specified and lawful purposes
- be processed in accordance with the person's rights under the DPA
- be adequate, relevant and not excessive in relation to that purpose
- be kept accurate and up-to-date
- not be kept for longer than is necessary for the given purpose
- be subject to appropriate safeguards against unauthorised use, loss or damage.

Q10. List three recommendations of the Caldicott Report.

The key recommendations are that the care worker must:
- justify a purpose for recording and using service user information
- only record and use information when it is absolutely necessary
- use only the minimum information required
- only access information on a strict 'need to know' basis
- be aware of their responsibilities concerning the recording and use of service user information
- understand and comply with the law eg. the Data Protection Act (1998).

CHAPTER THREE ANSWERS

Q1. What is ketosis?

The inefficient break down of fat caused by the absence of carbohydrates resulting in the production of ketones.

Q2. What are the symptoms of mild dehydration?

Feeling thirsty, dry mouth, concentrated urine, constipation, headaches, feeling tired

Q3. Why shouldn't you eat eggs after the 'best before' date?

Eggs can contain *Salmonella* bacteria, which could multiply to high levels if you keep them after this date.

Q4. What points should you remember when using cling flim?

Do not use cling film if it could melt into the food, such as in the oven or on pots and pans on the hob. You can use some types of cling film in the microwave, but make sure that it doesn't touch the food. Only let cling film touch high fat foods when the instructions on the box say this is permissible.

Q5. How do you know when food is properly cooked?

Food should be steaming hot all the way through. Equipment such as cooking thermometers or temperature probes can also be used to check the temperature if they are available.

Q6. A serving of a fruit or vegetable is equal to..?

- One medium sized vegetable or fruit (such as an apple, orange or banana)
- Two small fruits (such as kiwi fruit or plums)
- 80g of fresh, frozen or canned fruits or vegetables
- 150ml fruit juice
- A tablespoon of dried fruit
- One bowl of green salad

Q7. What should the temperature of a fridge be set at?

It should be between 0°C and 5°C.

Q8. Milk is a processed food. True or false?

True. Milk is pasteurised to kill bacteria.

Q9. At what temperature should cooked food be served?

The food should reach a temperature of 70°C for more than two minutes in the middle or thickest part.

Q10. Bacteria are killed by freezing. True or false?

False. Bacteria are not destroyed by the freezing process. Rather, they are just dormant for the time that the food is frozen.

CHAPTER FOUR ANSWERS

Q1. What are the general requirements of the Health and Safety at Work Act (1974)?

- To protect all people who work in your premises and any other people who visit your workplace
- To protect the health, safety and welfare of all employees, whether they are full-time or part-time
- To protect all employees who may be exposed to risk in their workplace activity

Q2. Which local authority officer is responsible for ensuring compliance with the Food Safety Act (1990)?

The environmental health officer

Q3. Which food types are subject to temperature control?

- Cooked products and ready to eat products
- Dairy products
- Smoked or cured ready to eat meat and fish and some raw fish
- Fresh pasta and uncooked/partly cooked pasta and dough products

Q4. What is the Care Quality Commission?

The Care Quality Commission (CQC) is an independent agency set up by the government as a result of the Health and Social Care Act (2008). It promotes improvements and ensures quality standards are being met by social care services. It reports to government and publishes a report to parliament on the state of social care.

Q5. What do the CQC Essential Standards of Quality and Safety say about the use of menus?

Service users should have accessible information about meals and the arrangements for mealtimes. They should also have a choice for each meal that takes account of their individual preferences and needs, including their religious and cultural requirements.

Q6. List three factors that a food safety policy should cover.

- Food storage
- Food preparation
- Cleaning procedures
- Waste disposal
- Personal hygiene of staff
- Record keeping
- Staff training

Q7. List three things that a nutrition policy should cover.

- Nutritional needs assessment
- How to refer those who are at risk of malnutrition
- The minimum standards expected for the provision of food and drink
- How staff are introduced to and trained in good practice
- How eating and drinking records are maintained

Q8. What are protected mealtimes?

All non-urgent activity – such as drug rounds, tests etc – should be ceased during mealtimes. This allows service users to eat their meals without being interrupted by another activity and gives care staff the time to help those who need help eating. People must be given appropriate assistance when needed and sufficient time to eat their meals.

Q9. What is the 'red tray' system?

People who need help with eating should be identified on admission and a system put in place to signal the need for help. For example, serving their food on red (or different colour) trays allows staff to easily recognise those who need help at mealtimes.

Q10. What is of paramount importance in implementing a 'red tray' system?

That it works in practice – ie. that the service users receive the assistance they need to enable them to eat their meals and that their dignity is maintained.

Appendix B

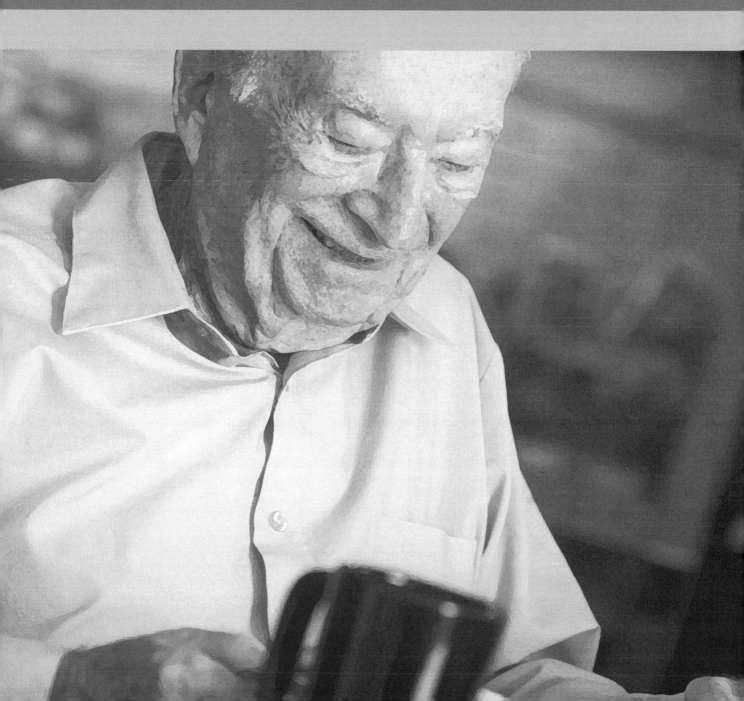

Sample nutrition policy

Aims of this policy

It is the aim of this organisation to provide service users with varied and nutritious meals that reflect individual food preferences and dietary needs.

Responsibilities

The home manager or the person in charge is responsible for ensuring that catering and care staff provide each individual with appropriate nutrition, according to individual preferences and needs.

The chef/cook is responsible for providing a menu that offers adequate nourishment and choice to cater for the needs of individuals, including those with specific nutritional needs.

The care and kitchen staff are responsible for ensuring that individuals are given a choice (with assistance if necessary) from the menu and that it is suitable for their individual nutritional requirements.

Nutritional assessment

Prior to admission, the home manager will have identified the nutritional needs of the service user in consultation with other relevant professionals.

Within 24 hours of admission, the person in charge will ensure that all residents are screened for risk of malnutrition using a validated nutrition screening tool such as MUST. If the initial assessment identifies risk of malnutrition an individual care plan will be drawn up according to the local nutrition policy/guidelines.

The person in charge will discuss the nutritional needs of the service user with the chef/cook.

The service user will be screened for risk of malnutrition using a validated nutrition screening tool such as MUST every four weeks or more frequently according to their individual condition.

Where a service user is found to be at risk of malnutrition, the local nutrition policy or guidelines should be followed. This may include providing nourishing snacks, nourishing drinks and food fortification. Service users at high risk of malnutrition may require referral to a dietitian.

Eating environment

The person in charge ensures that the eating environment is conducive to the enjoyment of meals. Service users have the opportunity to select meals from a varied menu that they can read and understand.

Furniture, napkins, cutlery and crockery that promote dignity, choice and independence are available and are used properly. Food is presented attractively and portions reflect the service user's individual appetite.

Individuals are offered a choice of drinks at regular intervals throughout the day to ensure their fluid intake is adequate.

Assistance is available to individuals who require help with eating and drinking. Individuals are encouraged to eat and drink at their own pace and there is no time limit placed on the meal.

Levels of background noise are kept to a minimum during mealtimes.

Medicine administration and GP visits are discouraged at mealtimes.

Family, friends and volunteers are welcomed at mealtimes and encouraged to eat with service users, or to assist individuals with their eating and drinking.

Provision of snacks and hot or cold drinks

Kitchen and care staff are responsible for ensuring that individuals have access to drinks and snacks throughout the day and night, according to their needs. Drinks and snacks are offered to all service users at mid-morning, mid-afternoon and early evening and before retiring to bed. Service users are able to request drinks and snacks at other times.

Service users are provided with a covered jug of fluid and tumbler, which are washed and replenished at breakfast, lunch and evening mealtimes.

To ensure that individuals have an adequate intake of fluids, all staff should be made aware that adults should aim to drink at least six to eight glasses of fluid in 24 hours. Therefore, drinks between meals should be encouraged.